Language Difficulties in an Educational Context

WENDY RINALDI, PhD, MRCSLT

Freelance Consultant in Child Communication and Learning

with contributions from

JAMES LAW PhD, *Lecturer, City University, London and*
JANET LARCHER PhD, *Freelance Consultant in Micro-technology Aids*

W

WHURR PUBLISHERS

LONDON AND PHILADELPHIA

© 2000 Whurr Publishers
First published 2000 by
Whurr Publishers Ltd
19b Compton Terrace, London N1 2UN, England and
325 Chestnut Street, Philadelphia PA 1906, USA
Except © Chapters 1, 3, 4, 5 – Wendy Rinaldi

British Library Cataloguing in Publication Data
A catalogue record for this book is available from the
British Library.

ISBN: 1 86156 156 3

Printed and bound in the UK by Athenaeum Press Ltd,
Gateshead, Tyne & Wear

Contents

Preface

This book's concept is underpinned by my experience of working as a language specialist in schools. My first job, in 1983, was split amongst many sites: a hospital, a health clinic, an assessment centre and a school. In that first job I approached working in education as a health service employee, very much from the medical perspective that I had gleaned from my student days. But I soon discovered that the 'find the root of the problem and fix it' notion of a medical model applied to hardly any of my work, whether in a health or school environment. Yes, I could try to alleviate problems, but the solution seemed to more closely resemble an educational process than a remedy. I also discovered that my contribution as a speech and language therapist was much more valued by parents, teachers and other professionals if I viewed communication beyond the communication process itself. After all, if I was to set about trying to develop a child's communication, why not do it in ways that would impact upon learning curriculum subjects or upon personal and social development? The links between communication, learning and social knowledge were much clearer than I expected; the effects much more far-reaching. It is this that inspired me to specialize in childhood language difficulties in education, to research, to publish my work and to teach others.

This book is a sharing of much that I have come to know in my journey through that educational process, with 'guest chapters' by Dr James Law and Dr Janet Larcher on the routes I have visited relatively briefly. It has been written for practitioners, across the professions, involved with language impaired children. It is anticipated that it will also be helpful to student practitioners who will want to know of the issues and possibilities when working with language impaired children in education before they enter the field. Chapters 1 to 3, in particular, also provide a number of indicators that may be of interest to those entering the field of research. I hope that Chapter 5 will further be helpful at policy level, in particular to assist Education Departments that are reorganizing provision across mainstream and special schools to more effectively meet the needs of language impaired children. Finally, I hope that the material is sufficiently digestible to be accessible to parents who seek a clearer understanding of their child's educational needs.

Wendy Rinaldi
April 2000

Introduction

The framework for *Language Difficulties in an Educational Context* is essentially one of two halves: the first three chapters are to do with concepts and issues underlying practice; the final three chapters focus more on practice itself.

The 'concepts and issues' section is dealt with quite broadly in Chapter 1, which takes in a range of content relating to childhood language difficulty. The issues and concepts covered in this chapter are by no means exhaustive: the author has drawn upon her experience as a trainer and lecturer to deal with the issues and questions most frequently raised by practitioners. Chapter 1 also aims to highlight the areas of common ground in the special needs spectrum, which can sometimes be overlooked in attempts to categorize different conditions. The rationale taken is that to appreciate areas of common ground it is first necessary to explore some of the ways language difficulties are currently described or categorized.

In Chapter 2, the range of content narrows and deepens to consider issues surrounding the preschool period. It may seem rather strange to include a chapter on preschool children in a book about education. However, the book views education in its broadest sense, and whilst other chapters focus more on the school context it is relevant also to consider issues pertinent to preschool children. One of the key issues in the early years concerns accurate identification: this issue clearly has implications not only for children's learning experiences in the early years but also for when they enter school. The effects of early intervention upon the needs of children in later years is also considered in this chapter.

The third chapter focuses upon perhaps one of the most challenging areas of practice in current times: the 'grey' area between language disorder and autism. This chapter aims firstly to give the reader a clearer understanding of the nature of difficulty in the overlapping contexts of autism and language disorder and the shift in balance within the sociocognitive-linguistic triangle which can lead to judgements of Asperger's syndrome, autism or developmental language disorder. Secondly, the chapter presents a potential way forward to more effective management. This chapter (and the subsequent two chapters) is based upon the author's own perspective and ideology. The literature is drawn upon to illustrate the background against which this ideology developed, along with observations of practice. In some instances the author has needed to rely upon experience of practice to raise potentially important issues which could be subjected to research scrutiny.

The second half: 'Practice', starts in Chapter 4 by detailing an approach to develop language, learning and social behaviour in children across a range of special needs groups. The links between language, learning and social development first raised in Chapter 1 are built upon in this chapter by showing how a language-based approach can impact upon curriculum subjects and social times. There is first an overview to the rationale and key elements of a language-based approach, narrowing to the specifics of activities.

Chapter 5 then considers ways of implementing a language-based approach in both special and mainstream schools and culminates in the presentation of a model of inclusive education.

Finally, Chapter 6 focuses upon the use of information technology (IT) as a further medium in the delivery of a language-based approach. Although it is little explored in the literature on childhood language disorder, this chapter aims to show the potentially significant contribution that IT could make, within a repertoire of resources, to deliver a language-based approach when educating children with special needs.

Chapter 1
Perspectives on children with language difficulties

WENDY RINALDI

Introduction

Developmental language difficulty, in its various forms, cuts across the spectrum of special educational need. For example, a language difficulty is part of the picture of disability in learning difficulties, autism, Asperger's syndrome and sensory impairments. In addition, there is a group of children said to have **specific or primary** developmental language disorder, whose profile of abilities and skills has been identified as distinct from the aforementioned groups (Warnock, 1978; Emerick and Hatten, 1979; Rapin and Allen, 1983; Lees and Urwin, 1997).

Law et al.'s 1998 review of studies into the prevalence of speech and language difficulties between the ages of 2 to 5, quotes a median of 5% across studies. Albritton (1984) found 7% prevalence in students aged 12–13. However, this must be a vast underestimate when all children with language difficulties, across the special needs groups are considered: to coin a phrase there are 'so many out there'. Yet despite this, a debate surrounds basic issues such as: *What do we call these children? How can we best describe their difficulties? Are specific language difficulties another kind of specific learning difficulty? Which children can benefit from specialist intervention?*

Practitioners can sometimes feel a sense of frustration in wrangling over these issues in their search for practical solutions to enable children to learn to the best of their abilities. However, exploring these questions gives a better understanding of children's difficulties and can inform practice. For example, areas of common ground may be seen among the special needs groups and this can facilitate more effective management; describing children's language is usually the key to education planning and helps to explain the difficulties underpinning problems with learning or behaviour.

1

This chapter will thus begin to address these fundamental issues as a basis for focusing in more detail on aspects of education relevant to children with language difficulties in later chapters. In the main it draws upon the literature and upon research-based evidence; the author also includes some practice-based observations.

The name game: terminology for children with primary language difficulties

A variety of different terms are used to describe children who have a primary language difficulty. Earlier citations refer to 'developmental dysphasia' (Wyke, 1978; Rapin and Allen, 1983). Current literature refers to specific language impairment (SLI) or specific developmental language disorder (SDLD),[1] by those who wish to emphasize the developmental nature of the condition. The use of 'impairment' in the first term avoids the potential confusion between the abbreviations for specific language difficulties and severe learning difficulties.

The move away from the term developmental dysphasia occurred perhaps because the term dysphasia (partial impairment of language function) is used to describe acquired language disorder following, for example, stroke or brain injury. There are fundamental differences between acquired and developmental forms of language disorder; for example, in acquired forms there is a clearly identified etiology, whereas in developmental forms there is not. Aram and Eisele (1994) conclude that the type of unilateral neurological lesion to the left hemisphere, clearly identified in acquired childhood language disorders, cannot account for the persistent nature of language difficulty in SDLD.

Further terminology to describe types of language difficulty is discussed later in this chapter.

So what can account for specific developmental language difficulties?

Lees and Urwin (1997) characterize earlier attempts to define specific developmental language disorder as having been reached by exclusion: that is, there are no precipitating factors or predisposing factors to account for the language difficulty, such as those found in other special needs groups (e.g. sensory impairment, cognitive delay, etc.). However, Lees and Urwin observe that in fact the vast majority of SDLD children show certain precipitating or predisposing factors, or at least they have a

---

[1] In this book, the term specific developmental language disorder (SDLD) will be used.

history of such factors. Bishop (1992) also suggests a multifactorial etiology, where specific language difficulty is the final common pathway for a number of factors which interrupt development. Lees and Urwin therefore suggest a definition which acknowledges that a specific language disorder may be associated with a history of hearing, learning, environmental or emotional difficulty, but cannot be attributed to any one of these alone or even to the sum of these effects. That is, the precipitating factors are not present to a degree sufficient to bring about the degree of language disorder. Needless to say, whilst such a definition is conceptually helpful, the practicalities of deciding whether or not the associated difficulties could bring about the degree of language disorder may prove problematic in some cases and be very open to interpretation.

Lees and Urwin further outline four common findings seen in SDLD children. These are: a) a family history of specific difficulty with language; b) evidence of cerebral dysfunction, for example, presence of neurological signs such as clumsiness or epilepsy (Robinson, 1987); c) mismatches in the subsystems of language in relation to aspects of cognitive development and d) failure to catch up these differences with 'generalized' language stimulation. Kirchner and Skarakis-Doyle (1983) also assume a genetic or lesion-based disruption in the growth of language skills required for the development of normal communication. Lees and Urwin note, however, that despite their findings outlined in their points a) and b), as yet it has not proved possible to isolate a genetic marker for language disorder or to find evidence of clear cerebral lesions (Robinson, 1992). Nevertheless, over the past decade evidence has mounted to suggest an important genetic contribution in cases of SDLD (Tallal et al., 1989; Lewis and Thompson, 1992; Tomblin and Buckwater, 1994; Bishop et al., 1995; Lahey and Edwards, 1995; Bishop et al., 1999). Aram and Eisele (1994) suggest that any neurological basis of SDLD would be in terms of bilateral or diffuse areas of the brain.

Lees and Urwin's reference to mismatches in the subsystems of language in relation to cognitive development, may provide a way of differentiating specific language difficulties from those seen in moderate learning difficulties. The definition of SDLD usually includes average or above average ability on performance (non-language-based) IQ subtests. However, there are a group of children who score below average on performance subtests whilst demonstrating even greater difficulty on verbal IQ subtests or other standardized language assessments (Rinaldi, 1992). These children have moderate learning difficulties, but there is a specificity to their language difficulty because of the mismatches in the language profile in relation to cognitive development. Other children with moderate learning difficulties do not show these mismatches.

Cromer (1987) highlights the importance of underlying perceptual and cognitive impairments to account for SDLD, in particular those affecting auditory processing and memory. For example, Tallal and Piercy (1973, 1978), and Tallal et al. (1981) found that 5–8-year-old SDLD children's ability to process the order of auditory signals was particularly affected by the rate of presentation. The younger children in their samples also had difficulty in processing visual stimuli. Considering memory, Menyuk (1978) found that SDLD children omitted the first part of sentences in repetition tasks. Gathercole and Baddley (1990) found that children with language difficulties performed less well than a group matched for vocab- ulary and reading skills on a task requiring immediate recall of non-words. Van der Lely and Howard (1993), however, did not find short-term memory deficits in verbal repetition and picture pointing tasks in a group of six SDLD children. They conclude that different groups of language impaired children may have different characteristics in short-term memory tasks. This variation in characteristics across sub-groups of language impairment may also be evident in auditory processing abilities. Frumkin and Rapin (1980) found that children with phonological difficulties were affected by the rate of presentation in auditory discrimination tasks, whereas language impaired children with normal phonology were not.

Bishop's (1992) pursuit of the difficulties underlying SDLD develops the earlier thinking of Menyuk, Tallal and Piercy. Whilst noting that a single underlying factor is unlikely to explain adequately all cases of SDLD, she proposes that a fundamental deficit may be a slowed rate of information processing leading to impairment in any task requiring integration of rapidly presented information. Bishop suggests that SDLD children may be able to perform normally on non-language-based tasks that require information processing, such as block design, because these tasks require them to use mental representations that are processed simultaneously. That is, all the necessary information for solving the task is present simultaneously and the individual blocks can be mentally manipulated into a single spatial represen- tation. However, the information processing deficit may show itself when the child has to process information that is transient, or when a transient repre- sentation must be held in mind while another representation is formed.

In the same paper, Bishop also explores the hypothesis that abnormal learning strategies may underlie SDLD. Her review focuses on hypothesis- testing abilities, and she concludes that this strategy does not appear to be deficient in SDLD children. However, it can be envisaged that difficulty with verbal learning strategies, such as requesting clarification or interjec- tion to check understanding, may influence the information processing capabilities of children. Guilford (1988) observed problems with requesting clarification in language impaired adolescents. Brinton and

Fujiki (1982) found that SDLD children made fewer requests for clarification than non-impaired children.

Cromer (1983) proposed that SDLD children may have difficulty in hierarchical planning and that this may underlie problems of language structure. He found that SDLD children were less likely than deaf children to use hierarchical planning when asked to copy hierarchical patterns; unfortunately, the groups were not matched on verbal skills so the causal relation between language ability and task performance is not clear. However, the idea that language impaired children may have difficulties appreciating the hierarchical nature of language may be worth pursuing. The author has noted that language impaired children, across special needs groups, appear not to appreciate the hierarchical relationship between word meanings; for example the relationship between category words with words belonging to categories. Rinaldi (1998, 1999) has found that categorization can be taught to children as a strategy for improving word finding and organizational language ability. Crystal (1987) also proposes categorization (hyponymy) as one of four word relationships that enable children to appreciate the structure of semantic fields.

Finally, it should be noted that deficits of language can *contribute* to poor performance on cognitive tasks. Even so-called non-verbal tasks such as visual memory recall may actually be assisted by linguistic strategies. For example, semantic associations may be used to recall visual symbols. Therefore, it may be envisaged that some SDLD children's ability on performance IQ subtests may be affected by their language difficulty and this could reduce the likelihood of a discrepancy between verbal and non-verbal IQ.

In summary, there appears to be some variation according to the nature of cognitive deficits which can be associated with SDLD, which is perhaps hardly surprising bearing in mind the heterogeneous nature of the disorder. However, there appears sufficient evidence to support Menyuk's (1978) claim that although SDLD children may attain values equivalent to average or above average intelligence on performance (non-language-based) IQ subtests, it is not true that these children are, except for language, cognitively intact.

The jury is still out on the question of how best to account for language disorders, however conclusions currently drawn favour a genetically determined deficit in cognitive processing. Bishop et al. (1999) raise the need to specify the underlying cognitive mechanisms that lead to SDLD and to understand which aspects of language processing are subject to genetic influence. Their study of a sample of children drawn from 141 twin pairs found no evidence of a heritable influence on auditory processing impairment. However, the study did reveal high estimates of group heritability in phonological short-term memory. Whilst identifying a genetic contribution to specific language disorders, this study also identifies the role of the environment and supports the view that environmental input may play a role in maintaining or facilitating problems. However, it is now generally accepted that environmental input does not *create* language disorders.

Specific language disorder: another kind of specific learning difficulty?

A related issue surrounding the notion of specific developmental language difficulty is whether or not this should be considered a form of specific learning difficulty.

This issue arises in part because of the related cognitive dysfunctions already identified in this chapter, and in part because there is clearly a learning element to children's acquisition of language. For example, young children make mistakes in learning linguistic rules. They can overgeneralize rules of grammar (for example the overuse of regular past tense forms 'ed' in 'runned', 'goed' etc.) and meaning (for example the use of the word 'dog' to apply to all four-legged animals). Children's questioning of figurative language and their use of context to learn new idiomatic meanings (Cacciari and Levorato, 1989) also suggest a conscious learning process in the later stages of communication development. It has therefore been proposed that SDLD should be considered a form of specific learning difficulty, as are specific difficulties with number and written language (Dockrell and McShane, 1993). The argument for some innate predisposition for language development (Chomsky, 1969, 1975; Butterworth, 1999) is, however, also attractive in accounting for the rapidity with which very young children acquire language. Butterworth's view is that 'children start off with little starter kits' (he extends this notion to numeracy also).

The relationship between specific difficulties in spoken and written language has been highlighted in recent years. Catts (1989, 1996) and Kamhi and Catts (1989) claim that many cases of dyslexia can best be defined as a developmental language disorder. Children with specific spoken language difficulties can also experience difficulties in written language, but not in every case. Stackhouse (1982) notes that not all children with spoken language difficulties will go on to have written difficulties. It is also the author's experience that children with a history of phonological disorder in the preschool years, who receive therapy to increase phonological awareness and use, can go on to become excellent readers when they enter school. A longitudinal study by Stothard et al. (1998), however, indicates the need for caution in interpreting literacy skills in children with a history of language impairment. Children whose language difficulties had resolved at age 5;6 showed no difficulty with reading and spelling at age 8;6 (Bishop and Adams, 1990). However, the same children showed weaker literacy skills than their peer group at 15–16 years. Stothard et al. therefore propose 'a protracted period of illusory recovery'. They speculate:

> the early acquisition of phonological awareness is supported in children with speech–language impairments through the process of speech and language treatment. Later in the acquisition of reading, when there are perhaps heavier demands on a broader range of language processing skills, these children begin to develop difficulties (p. 417).

It is not clear at this stage whether the children who had weaker literacy skills at 15–16 years had had specific phonological difficulties in the early years or whether their difficulties had included deficiencies across the language profile.

Investigations into pinpointing which elements of spoken language difficulty may be related to written language difficulty have identified a number of possibilities including phonological awareness (Bradley and Bryant, 1983; Mann and Liberman, 1984), syntactic ability (Bishop and Adams, 1990; Mangusson and Nauclear, 1990; Menyuk et al., 1991), semantic ability (Menyuk et al. 1991) and performance on metaphonological tasks (Mangusson and Nauclear, 1990). Menyuk et al. found that measures of metalinguistic abilities (abilities to reflect consciously on the nature and properties of language) gave the strongest prediction of later reading achievement.

As more becomes known about the relationship between spoken and written language difficulties, one conclusion which may be reached is that the term specific developmental language disorder (or specific language impairment) applies equally well, as an umbrella term, to children whose language difficulties may be specific to the spoken and/or written modality(ies).

Describing language difficulties

A further issue concerns how to describe or categorize the language impairment itself. This issue applies to all language impaired children, including those whose language difficulty is specific or primary in nature and those whose language difficulty forms part of a developmental profile associated with a distinct etiology, condition or syndrome, such as hearing/visual impairment, autism or a more general cognitive delay.

Language difficulties are usually described according to the area(s) of language affected. Consideration is also given to whether the difficulty concerns use of language only (expressive difficulty) or comprehension and use (receptive difficulty). Those areas commonly included are phonology (use of speech sounds to signal meaning), grammar (including syntactic combinations of words, phrases, sentences and clauses; grammatical markers), semantics (word and sentence meaning) and pragmatic (meaning open to interpretation; selection and organization of language for communication; interactive skills of communication).[2]

Using these kinds of descriptions can be very useful in helping professionals to understand areas of common ground among the children they work with. For example, children with Asperger's syndrome, or mild autism, show marked difficulties with social communication/pragmatic aspects of language (Aarons and Gittens, 1998; Rinaldi, 1999). Many children with specific developmental language difficulty also have difficulty with pragmatic elements of language (Guilford, 1988; Rinaldi, 1996a; 1996b; 2000): these show themselves more clearly as earlier difficulties with phonology and syntax improve and as the reliance upon communication to get by socially becomes greater.

Children with visual impairment can develop language normally but have difficulty with social interactions. Stockley (1994) reports a lack of awareness of interactive communication skills; for example, one partially sighted student in her study commented: 'I didn't know people looked at each other when they talked'. Visually impaired students can also have difficulty in comprehending the meaning of non-verbal gestures such as facial expression and other forms of body language, because they have less experience of using and observing such gestures unless they are helped to focus upon them. Children with specific developmental language difficulty may also misinterpret non-verbal language, not through lack of experience, but because they do not appreciate the meaning of non-verbal forms unless this is specifically demonstrated.

A distinction between delay and disorder may also be made in describing children's language difficulty. Dockrell and McShane (1993) highlight potential problems in this distinction because of the variability in normal patterns of development. However, taking these variations into account, the idea of this distinction is that it is possible to determine whether or not a child's language is actually developing normally, albeit at a slower rate, with an indication that they will eventually 'catch up' with appropriate intervention. The term 'disorder' is indicative that the child's language is not developing normally and suggests the need for specialist intervention. In the following chapter, James Law will look at some of the considerations when making this distinction in early language development. In the school years the delay/disorder distinction appears to have little practical value, since although the child may appear to be using

---

[2] These areas will be dealt with more fully in Chapter 3, in clarifying the nature of pragmatic disorder, and in Chapter 4, in examining the relation between language and learning across the curriculum.

or understanding language at a stage appropriate for a much younger child, the indication is that they will not 'catch up' unless the difficulty is specifically addressed in teaching/therapy.

Language disorder sub-types: catalyst or constraint?

Within the field of specific developmental language difficulty there has been an attempt to develop sub-types of disorder. For example, one of the best known classifications in current use in the UK, based upon a large empirical study, is that of Rapin and Allen (1987). This classification includes phonologic–syntactic disorder (severe phonological problems accompanied by grammatical deficits); lexical–syntactic disorder (severe word-finding difficulties, immature syntax, but normal phonology) and semantic–pragmatic disorder (particular difficulties with encoding meaning relevant to the conversational situation; fluent complex speech with clear articulation).

Attempts to categorize language disorders in this way can be seen as practically helpful in that, because they list a number of features, they enable a relatively swift decision to be made on the nature of difficulty. However, the heterogeneity of language disorders may mean that a classification system based on sub-types is too narrow and, therefore, limiting. The American Speech/Language Association's (1980) definition of SDLD identifies that the disorder may involve all of the phonologic, syntactic, semantic or pragmatic elements of the linguistic subsystem. Dockrell and McShane (1989) observe that most SDLD children exhibit a pattern of difficulty across several language components. Similarly, Rinaldi (1996a) cites evidence of children whose difficulties occur across all language areas (phonology, grammar, semantics/lexicon and pragmatics) and whose profiles change as they develop through the school years. Rinaldi (2000) has also shown that pragmatic and semantic difficulties do not necessarily co-occur.

A further disadvantage of applying a classification system such as Rapin and Allen's is that it suggests that the language picture seen in SDLD may be different from that seen in other special needs groups. As has already been indicated, this may be a false picture. The differences between SDLD children, as a group, and children who have language difficulty forming part of a broader picture of special needs, may be less to do with the observed language difficulty and more to do with factors underpinning the difficulty concerning, for example, cognitive or perceptual ability.

Deficits underpinning difficulties in the subsystems of language (phonology, syntax, semantics, pragmatics) and their interactions have been explored by psycholinguistic models (for example, Butterworth, 1980; Dockrell and McShane, 1993; Stackhouse and Wells, 1993).

Stackhouse and Wells' model, originally developed to assess developmental disorders of speech, proposes levels of breakdown at input, output
and internal representation. Such levels of breakdown can provide a
useful concept in exploring language difficulties[3] because whereas, for
example, some children have difficulty in processing incoming information, others can actually process the information but then have difficulty in
dealing with or acting upon the information appropriately. That is, the
information goes in and registers, but once this has happened children
'don't know where to go with it'. Skills needed at the level of internal
representation are likely to include those already referred to in this
chapter, such as metalinguistic/metacommunicative knowledge, the ability
to process transient information (Bishop, 1992), hierarchical planning,
mechanisms to store and retrieve information, etc.

The teaching approach described in Chapter 4 attempts to address
potential breakdown at different levels of processing including, for
example, adjustments to inputs, strategies for accessing incoming information, strategies for more effective internal representation and use or
'output' of information to demonstrate learning and communicate
socially.

Interestingly, it has been the author's experience that, given a language-
based approach to teaching, children from different special needs groups
can learn well together, despite the differing factors underpinning their
difficulties. It is their rate and, to some extent, their style of learning that
varies. This will be discussed further in Chapters 3, 4 and 5.

From primary to secondary school

It is now fairly well documented that the picture of language disorder
changes as the child develops through primary to secondary school
(Griffiths, 1969; Aram and Nation, 1975; Guilford, 1988; Ehren and Lenz,
1989). The learning and social demands upon children also change.

Griffiths (1969) found that children who had apparently overcome
their oral language difficulties in the primary years were having continuing
education and social problems at secondary school. Stothard et al. (1998)
found that children whose language problems had resolved at age 5;6
performed significantly less well at 15–16 years than non-impaired peers
on tests of phonological processing and literacy skills. There were no
differences between the groups on tests of vocabulary and
semantic/grammatical comprehension. However, tests of pragmatic

---

[3] Breakdown in levels of pragmatic processing will be referred to in more detail in
Chapter 3.

language were not included and, as will be shown in subsequent paragraphs, this aspect of language may be an area of vulnerability in secondary school students with a history of language difficulty.

In the study by Stothard et al., children whose language problems had not resolved by age 5;6 continued to have difficulty at 15–16 years and the authors conclude:

> If a child's language difficulties are still present at age 5;6 ... the child will be at a high risk of language, literacy and educational difficulties throughout childhood and adolescence. In contrast, if the child's language difficulties are largely resolved by 5;6, then the outlook for spoken language is better. However, although none of the children in this subgroup (at 15–16 years) would meet criteria for developmental dyslexia, their literacy skills were weak in relation to their peer group(p. 417).

It is argued in this book that the outlook and need for future specialist help, in children whose language difficulties appear to have resolved either before or shortly after school entry, cannot be accurately assessed unless pragmatic language/communication skills are examined. This view is endorsed by Aram and Nation's (1975) report that as language disordered children grow older, the language disorder becomes more specific, and by the observations of Guilford (1988), which emphasize the area of pragmatics. For example, Guilford describes a tendency for adolescent language impaired students to be less sensitive to conversational rules and to show a disinclination to request clarification when given an ambiguous message by peers. Rinaldi (2000) identified particular difficulties with pragmatic comprehension for 11 to 14-year-old SDLD children.

In Chapter 4 the areas of semantics and pragmatics will be identified as central to accessing curriculum subjects; the area of pragmatics is also central to social development. Indeed, although the nature of language disorder can, in a sense, become more specific in later years, as earlier difficulties with phonology and syntax lessen, Ehren and Lenz note that, because of changes in school demand, the effect of the language disorder manifests itself more broadly in terms of curriculum areas and therefore may be mislabelled as a learning difficulty: 'As these students mature, the language disorders at the root of their difficulties in school are often forgotten as the label of "language disordered" is traded for another educational tag, more often than not "learning disabled".'(p. 193).

The curriculum offered at secondary school is not only broader than that at primary school but the depth of learning in each subject also requires the comprehension of increasingly abstract language concepts. There is also a need to understand and use specialized vocabulary not in frequent use and thus more difficult to remember. Further, as children grow older they are expected to plan and organize language in more creative tasks, such as essay writing, developing projects, interpreting literature and artwork. Social communication becomes increasingly important in friendship: chat, jokes, sending notes and so on.

The more abstract nature of learning makes subjects harder to teach through multisensory methods, which include visual and experiential learning to supplement auditory inputs. However, this approach is vital for language impaired children: difficulty with auditory elements of processing and memory render the auditory input channel the weakest.

Ehren and Lenz (1989) identify two distinct groups within the adolescent language disordered population: a) those who have a history of language disorder identified in the primary school years and whose problem persists, albeit with changing symptoms, and b) those whose language disorder manifested itself in more subtle ways when they were younger and have only become observable as the demands of the school context require a greater reliance on language competence.

It also has to be borne in mind that some language skills develop later. For example, the comprehension of ambiguous meaning, normally develops around the age of 7 to 10 years (Ackerman, 1982; Cacciari and Levorato, 1989; Rotenburg et al., 1989). It is at this age that children are expected to understand such communication and it is at this age therefore that difficulties here will show themselves. For example, reading and television material aimed at junior and secondary school children assumes understanding of figurative language and sarcasm. Nippold (1991) found that in three reading programmes developed for 8 to 13-year-olds, an idiom occurred in 6.7% of all sentences. Lazar et al. (1989) found that, on average, 11% of teachers' utterances in class groups of 11-year-olds contained at least one idiom; this figure rose to 20% for teachers talking to 13-year-olds.

Damico (1988) also emphasizes the importance of considering the changing demands upon children that reveal difficulties which are not apparent when the child enters primary school. He studied a 12-year-old who had received speech and language therapy and was discharged, reportedly having acceptable speech and language production. However, the child continued to have difficulties at home and school and a later assessment identified language difficulties that were not apparent earlier.

In summary, the study by Stothard et al. (1998) indicates a brighter outlook for children whose language difficulties are resolved by age 5;6, endorsing the importance of early intervention. However, the message underlying findings of other studies reported in this chapter is that even when specific help is given to children in the early years of development, it is quite possible that they will continue to need help as they grow older.

This may be so even if their language development is 'within normal limits' when they enter primary school. Damico (1988) calls for further long-term follow-up of children who have marked speech and language disorders in early life; it is proposed in this book that a crucial element of follow-up is the assessment of pragmatic language/communication skills. The long-term follow-up of children may appear a considerable task and emphasizes the importance of research identifying criteria that will indicate which children are likely to have difficulties in later life (Enderby and Emerson, 1995). This line of inquiry will be referred to again in Chapter 2; it should, however, be noted that for children who have specific difficulties with the elements of language acquired in the later stages of development, there may not be any indications early on in life. The necessity for school special needs coordinators to be alert to these kinds of difficulties is highlighted here.

Specificity: should it determine the level of specialist intervention?

It has been acknowledged (Warnock, 1978) that children with specific developmental language difficulties require special means of access to the curriculum. This 'access' is usually provided by speech and language therapists and/or specialist teachers who have knowledge in language disorder, gained through experience and postgraduate training. An increasing number of teachers are gaining specialist qualifications in language difficulties, although at the time of writing this is not compulsory.

The language needs of children from other special needs groups has been less clearly identified. The amount of speech and language therapy available to these children, for example, is usually much smaller than that available to children with specific difficulties. Statements of educational need may include 'speech and language therapy advice/monitoring', suggesting that the child will not have direct contact with a speech and language therapist or language specialist teacher. Wording may be included to indicate that the language difficulty forms part of a more 'global' difficulty.

The implication may be that the child's language skills will develop alongside other developmental skills, such as those of cognition, motor development, etc., without being specifically addressed through teaching. The educational approach available to these children may therefore include adjustment to take into account the pace or level of learning, but may not include a language focus. However, it is the author's experience that language can provide a 'window' into learning for children with special needs, regardless of the specificity of the difficulty. That is, the specialist, language-based approach, identified as being required for children with specific language difficulties, may be equally applicable across special needs groups.

Case study data (Rinaldi, unpublished) shows that children who may initially be described, on the basis of IQ scores, as having moderate learning difficulties can, with language-based learning, progress to 'within the average range'. It will be further argued, in Chapter 5, that elements of the approach to facilitate learning among special needs children may also accelerate mainstream children's learning.

The impact of language difficulties and language-based education

A language difficulty is more than simply a language difficulty; this is so because language is central to living. Language is used not only to communicate, but also to learn. Children also need it to develop socially: to make and sustain friendships. A rare longitudinal study by Haynes and Naidoo (1991) into how language impaired children fare when they leave school, emphasizes the social impact of language difficulties. They found that in a sample of 34 SDLD students followed up at 18 and 22 years, many had difficulty with social interaction. Although 20 of the 34 students reported going out socially with friends of their own age, 14 of the 20 did so only rarely. Fujiki et al. (1996) also found SDLD children to have poorer social skills, fewer peer relationships and to be less satisfied with peer relationships than age-matched classmates.

Figures 1.1 and 1.2 (revised from Rinaldi, 1996a) summarize some of the ways in which a child with language difficulties can be disadvantaged in learning and social contexts.

A further impact of language difficulty may be to create behaviour that is difficult to manage. It may be proposed that all children with special needs are vulnerable to low self esteem as they become more aware of the difficulties they have in relation to others. Low self esteem is also commonly at the heart of disruptive or withdrawn behaviour. The work of Dreikurs (1995), emanating from the psychology of Adler, identifies that attention-seeking, aggressive or revengeful behaviour can develop if children do not feel valued in the family group. His view is that this behaviour is the result of the child actually trying to find an identity or 'place' within their family, but going about it in the wrong way and thus creating feelings of irritation, anger or hurt in others. Dreikurs views withdrawn behaviour as the child 'giving up', and notes that this creates feelings of helplessness in the family. It could be envisaged that these patterns of behaviour (referred to as 'mistaken goals' by Dreikurs) may also emerge as a result of the child's sense of his or her value within the peer group or in the broader school context.

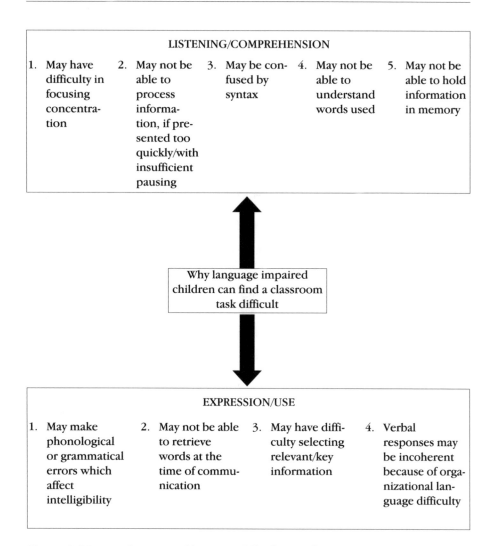

Figure 1.1 Potential impacts of language difficulties on learning.

The 'mistaken goals' form a starting point for helping children to see alternative ways of achieving their desired aim.[4]

In addition to effects on self esteem, there are other ways in which a language difficulty can more specifically create behaviour that can be difficult to manage. These are summarized in Figure 1.3.

Figures 1.1 to 1.3 may appear to present rather a bleak picture, but from another perspective they project a very positive one, because just as a

---

[4] Beattie (1996) has more recently developed literature for parents and professionals, based upon the work of Adler and Dreikurs (Dreikurs, 1995).

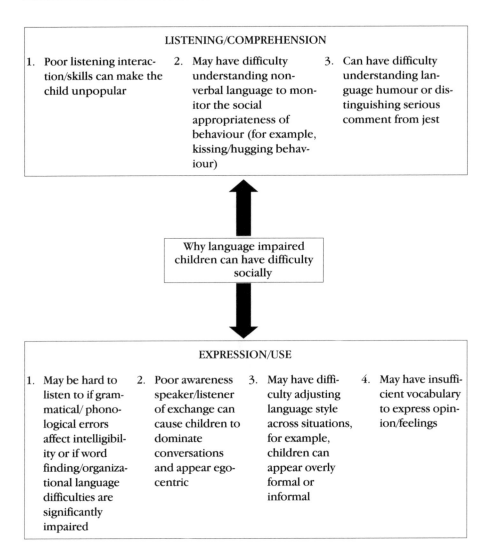

Figure 1.2 Potential impacts of language difficulties on social development.

difficulty with language may create learning and social difficulties, progress in the relevant language areas also creates progress in learning and social development. Similarly, behavioural difficulties can lessen as a result of focusing directly upon the language/communication skills underpinning the problematic behaviour.

Chapters 4 and 5 identify how a language/communication focus in education can be achieved with school-aged children, from nursery/infant through to secondary school.

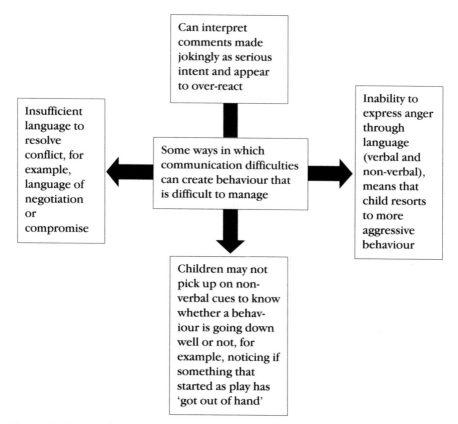

Figure 1.3 Potential impacts of language difficulties on behaviour.

Summary

- The area of language provides a focus for viewing areas of common ground among children with special needs.
- The etiology of SDLD remains hazy. A number of associated factors have been observed, but these do not always apply. The case for considering some kind of cognitive deficit relating to (but not necessarily causing) the language disorder appears strong, but the nature of deficit appears to vary according to the nature of the language difficulty. An underlying information-processing deficit of the kind described by Bishop (1992) may explain discrepancies between non-verbal (block design) and verbal IQ sub-tests. In the past decade evidence has grown for an important genetic contribution and a need for further study into which aspects of language/cognitive processing are subject to genetic influence has been identified.

- A language focus to education provides access to learning for all children with special needs; this approach is currently more likely to be offered to SDLD children only. There may also be an impact on social and personal development if an emphasis is placed on the elements of language that underpin social communication, peer relationships and/or problematic behaviour.
- The increasing demands upon language both in social and learning contexts are such that some children who enter primary school with language 'within normal limits' may show communication difficulties in later development.

The next chapter extends some of these themes, examining those issues particularly pertinent to the preschool period.

References

Aarons M, Gittens T. Autism: A Social Skills Approach. Oxford: Winslow Press, 1998.

Ackerman B. On comprehending idioms: do children get the picture? Journal of Experimental Psychology 1982; 33: 439–54.

Albritton T. Secondary speech-language programs: strategies for a new delivery system. Paper presented at the annual convention of the American Speech–Hearing Association, San Francisco, 1984.

Aram DM, Eisele J. Limits to a left hemispheric explanation for specific language impairment. Journal of Speech and Hearing Research 1994; 37: 824–30.

Aram D, Nation JE. Patterns of language behaviour in children with developmental disorders. Journal of Speech and Hearing Research 1975; 18: 229–41.

Beattie L. Tips in Discipline with Children (4th edition). Aylesbury: Adlerian Workshops and Publications, 1996.[5]

Bishop DVM. The underlying nature of specific language impairment. Journal of Child Psychology and Psychiatry 1992; 33: 3–66.

Bishop DVM, Adams C. A prospective study of the relationship between specific language impairment, phonological disorders and reading retardation. Journal of Child Psychology and Psychiatry 1990; 31 (7): 1027–50.

Bishop DVM, Bishop SJ, Bright P, James C, Delaney T and Tallal P. Different origin of auditory and phonological processing problems in children with language impairment: evidence from a twin study. Journal of Speech and Hearing Research 1999; 42: 155–68.

Bloom L, Lahey M. Language Development and Language Disorders. London: John Wiley and Sons, 1978.

Bradley L, Bryant P. Categorising sounds and learning to read: a causal connexion. Nature 1983; 301: 419–21.

[5] Training courses are also available from Adlerian Workshops and Publications, 216 Tring Rd, Aylesbury, Bucks.

Brinton B, Fujiki M. A comparison of request–response sequences in the discourse of normal and language-disordered children. Journal of Speech and Hearing Disorders 1982; 47: 57–62.

Brinton B, Fujiki M, Winkler E, Loeb D. Responses to requests for clarification in linguistically normal and language-impaired children. Journal of Speech and Hearing Disorders 1986; 51: 370–8.

Butterworth B. A model of speech production. Unpublished lecture, University College, London, Psychology Dept, 1980.[6]

Butterworth B. True grit (opinion). New Scientist July 1999.

Cacciari C, Levorato M. How children understand idioms in discourse. Journal of Child Language 1989; 16: 387–405.

Catts HW. Defining dyslexia as a developmental language disorder. Annals of Dyslexia 1989; 39: 50–64.

Catts HW. Defining dyslexia as a developmental language disorder: an expanded view. Topics in Language Disorders 1996; 16: 14–29.

Chomsky N. The Acquisition of Syntax in Children from 5 to 10. Cambridge, MA: MIT Press, 1969.

Chomsky N. Reflections on Language. Cambridge, MA: MIT Press, 1975.

Cromer R. Hierarchical planning disability in the drawings and constructions of a group of severely dysphasic children. Brain and Cognition 1983; 2: 144–64.

Crystal D. Concept of language development: a realistic perspective. In Rule R, Rutter M (eds), Language Development and Language Disorders. London: MacKeith Press, 1987.

Damico JS. The lack of efficacy in language therapy: a case study. Language, Speech and Hearing Services in Schools 1988; 19: 41–50.

Dockrell J, McShane J. Children's Learning Difficulties: A Cognitive Approach. Oxford: Blackwell, 1993.

Dreikurs R. Happy Children. Melbourne: Australian Council for Educational Research Ltd, 1995.

Ehren B, Lenz B. Adolescents with language disorders: special considerations in providing academically relevant language intervention. Seminars in Speech and Language 1989; 10: 192–204.

Emerick L, Hatten J. Diagnosis and Evaluation in Speech Pathology. Englewood Cliffs, NJ: Prentice Hall, 1979.

Enderby P, Emerson J. Does Speech and Language Therapy Work? London: Whurr Publishers Ltd, 1995.

Frumkin B, Rapin I. Perception of vowels and consonant-vowels of varying duration in language-impaired children. Neuropsychologia, 1980; 18: 443–54.

Fujiki M, Brinton B, Todd C. Social skills of children with specific language impairment. Language, Speech and Hearing Services in Schools 1996; 27: 195–201.

---

[6] Butterworth's model is included, with kind permission from the author, in Rinaldi (1997), Understanding Pragmatic Meaning. A Study of Secondary School Students with Specific Developmental Language Disorders. PhD Thesis, held at London University, Institute of Education Library.

Gathercole S, Baddley A. Phonological memory deficits in language-disordered children: is there a causal connection? Journal of Memory and Language 1990; 29: 336–60.

Griffiths C. A follow up study of children with articulation and language disorders. British Journal of Disorders of Communication 1969; 4: 46–56.

Guilford A. Language disorders in the adolescent. In Lass N, McReynolds L, Northern J, Yoder D. (eds) Handbook of Speech-Language and Pathology. Toronto: BC Decker, 1988.

Haynes C, Naidoo S. Children with specific speech and language impairment. Clinics in Developmental Medicine 119. London: MacKeith Press, 1991.

Kamhi A, Catts HW. Reading Disabilities: A Developmental Language Perspective. Boston, MA: Allyn & Bacon, 1989.

Kirchner D, Skarakis-Doyle E. Developmental language disorders: a theoretical perspective. In Gallagher T, Prutting C (eds), Pragmatic Assessment and Intervention Issues in Language. San Diego, CA: College Hill Press, 1983.

Law J, Boyle J, Harris F, Harkness A. Child Health Surveillance: Screening for Speech and Language Delay. Monograph published by the NHS Centre for Reviews and Dissemination, University of York, 1998.

Lazar RT, Warr- Leeper GA, Nicholson CB, Johnson S. Elementary school teachers' use of multiple meaning expressions. Language, Speech and Hearing Services in Schools 1989; 20: 240–50.

Lees J, Urwin S. Children with Language Disorders. London: Whurr Publishers Ltd, 1997.

Mangusson E, Nauclear K. Reading and spelling in language-disordered children: linguistic and metalinguistic prerequisites. Report on a longitudinal study. Clinical Linguistics and Phonetics 1990; 4: 49–61.

Mann V, Liberman I. Phonological awareness and verbal short term memory. Journal of Learning Disabilities 1984; 17: 592–9.

Menyuk P. Linguistic problems in children with developmental dysphasia. In Wyke M (ed) Developmental Dysphasia. London: Academic Press, 1978.

Menyuk P, Chesnik M, Libergott JW, Korngold B, D'Agostino R, Belanger A. Predicting reading problems in at-risk children. Journal of Speech and Hearing Research 1991; 34: 893–903.

Nippold MA. Evaluating and enhancing idiom comprehension in language disordered students. Language, Speech and Hearing Services in Schools 1991; 22: 100–6.

Rapin I, Allen DA. Developmental language disorders: nosologic considerations. In Kirk U (ed) Neuropsychology of Language, Reading and Spelling. New York: Academic Press, 1983.

Rinaldi WF. Working with Language Impaired Teenagers with Moderate Learning Difficulties. London: I CAN, 1992.

Rinaldi WF. Understanding Ambiguity: An Assessment of Pragmatic Meaning Comprehension. Windsor: NFER-Nelson, 1996a.

Rinaldi WF. The inner life of youngsters with specific developmental language disorder. In Varma V (ed) The Inner Life of Children with Special Needs. London: Whurr Publishers Ltd, 1996b.

Rinaldi WF. Language Concepts to Access Learning. Guildford: Child Communication and Learning, 1998.

Rinaldi WF. Language Choices. Guildford: Child Communication and Learning, 1999.

Rinaldi WF. Pragmatic comprehension in secondary school aged students with specific developmental language disorder. International Journal of Language and Communication Disorders 2000; 35 (1): 1–29.

Robinson RJ. The causes of language disorder: introduction and overview. Proceedings of the First International Symposium of Specific Speech and Language Disorders in Children, Reading, Berks. London: AFASIC, 1987.

Robinson RJ. Brain imaging and language. In Fletcher P, Hall D (eds) Specific Speech and Language Disorders in Children. London: Whurr Publishers Ltd, 1992.

Rotenburg K, Simourd L, Moore D. Children's use of a verbal–non-verbal consistency principle to infer truth and lying. Child Development 1989; 60: 309–22.

Stackhouse J. An investigation of reading and spelling performance in speech-disordered children. British Journal of Disorders of Communication 1982; 17 (2): 53–60.

Stackhouse J, Wells B. Psycholinguistic assessment of developmental speech disorders. European Journal of Disorders of Communication 1993; 28 (4): 331–48.

Stockley J. Teaching social skills to visually impaired children. British Journal of Visual Impairment 1994; 12: 1.

Stothard SE, Snowling MJ, Bishop DVM, Chipchase BB, Kaplan CA. Language impaired pre-schoolers: a follow-up into adolescence. Journal of Speech, Language and Hearing Disorders 1998; 41: 407–18.

Tallal P, Piercy M. Developmental aphasia: impaired rate of non-verbal processing as a function of sensory modality. Neuropsychologia 1973; 11: 389–98.

Tallal P, Piercy M. Defects of auditory perception in children with developmental dysphasia. In Wyke M (ed), Developmental Dysphasia. London: Academic Press, 1978.

Tallal P, Ross R, Curtiss S. Familial aggregation in specific language impairment. Journal of Speech and Hearing Disorders 1989; 54: 167–73.

Tallal P, Stark R, Kallman C, Mellits D. A re-examination of some non-verbal perceptual abilities of language-impaired and normal children as a function of age and sensory modality. Journal of Speech and Hearing Research 1981; 24: 351–7.

Van der Lely HKJ, Howard D. Children with specific language impairment: linguistic impairment or short term memory deficit. Journal of Speech and Hearing Research 1993; 36: 1193–207.

Warnock M. Report on the Committee of Inquiry into the Education of Handicapped Children. London: HMSO, 1978.

Wyke M (ed) Developmental Dysphasia. London: Academic Press, 1978.

Chapter 2
Developmental language disorders: the preschool years

JAMES LAW

Introduction

Developmental language disorders often present a confusing picture to both practitioners and managers. In part this is a function of the range of different professionals who have been involved with language disordered children; all with their own professional languages and implied meanings. In part it is a function of the inherent complexity of a relatively new field, which has yet to be comprehensively mapped out. In this chapter I would like to review the current understanding of the concept of developmental language disorder and in particular pick out the identification of primary or what have come to be known as *specific* language impairments. I want to suggest that the present system of classification does not necessarily serve us particularly well and needs to be re-addressed as a dynamic synthesis of a number of closely related domains of the literature. Current arguments, particularly those related to the differential diagnosis of specific language impairment, may not be particularly relevant to setting priorities with the younger child: it may be more important to consider what we need to know if we are to provide appropriate support to children in the preschool period. This will encompass a broader conception of case status[1] and will emphasize the issue of prevention and whether it is possible to establish the relative risk of a child having a disorder which will go on to impact on subsequent performance.

The emphasis throughout this chapter will be on early stages of development, when language difficulties are often construed as a potential

---

[1] Case status refers to the identification of a child as being in need of specialist intervention, for example, beyond what would otherwise be available through the nursery/education system.

obstacle to wellbeing and psychological health. At this time, although the child will not yet have entered school, the process of education will have begun. Priorities are likely to change for children as they enter the education system. The needs of children as they progress through school, from nursery/infant through to secondary phases, are the subject of other chapters.

What is a developmental language disorder in the preschool years?

A developmental language disorder represents a significant deviation from the normal rate or pattern of language development in young children. For many children it is likely to be a persistent problem that can affect their educational attainment and social wellbeing. Such disorders can be very obvious, especially if they are associated with speech difficulties. But more often they go unrecognized or undetected by those around the child affected until well after the time when he or she would have been expected to start speaking. This concept of a deviation from the normal suggests that there is a useful concept of 'normality' from which it is possible to deviate, and that there is a unitary phenomenon known as 'language', which can be characterized in this way. Although it is possible to confine our understanding of language to specific aspects such as the production of morphemes, the use or comprehension of certain syntactic structures, the development of contextual meaning, or the production of narrative, it is clear that there is a wide range of linguistic phenomena which fall under the umbrella of language disorder. For many of these phenomena the normal sequence of development has been mapped out and can be found in many texts on the subject (see Adams et al., 1997 for a recent example). In the more severe cases difficulties in all these areas may co-occur, but it is likely that the child will have strengths in one area and weaknesses in others, as might be expected of a child with normally developing language.

However, the rate at which it is normal to acquire the necessary skills remains something of a moot point. Clearly there is a great deal of variation in children's language skills in the early years and this makes the issue of case definition particularly problematic. Some authors suggest that any deviation from a statistically derived norm is sufficient to determine whether a child has a language disorder. But such a definition relies on statistical convention related to the normal distribution and probably on measures that are often relatively insecure in psychometric terms. It also tends to lead to a rather sterile discussion of the value of identifying cases at –1 or –2 standard deviations below the norm on a given test. In practice, much of the description of developmental language disorders comes from extreme cases. At one level this is perfectly appropriate and leads to some very useful insights into the strengths and weaknesses of the individuals concerned. However, there has been a tendency to assume that any deviation from the statistical norm constitutes a language disorder. Therefore, as with any condition where there is a continuity of skills, there has been a tendency to identify an increasingly wide range of children. Exactly where the line should be drawn between normality and a clinical or special educational need remains unresolved for the present.

Specific or general language disorders?

For many years a distinction has been drawn between specific language difficulties and language difficulties that are associated with more general learning difficulties. This distinction may have some bearing on what sort of intervention[2] the children receive and is often favoured by parents who are adamant that their child is not experiencing general learning difficulties. The extent to which there is a theoretical rationale for such a position depends on one's view of language development. If it is assumed that language functions in a modular fashion, that it is a separate cognitive function which develops independently of other cognitive skills, such a separation of language as a discrete difficulty is relatively easy to explain. Indeed, specific language deficits may provide further rationale for the concept of a separate cognitive system (Pinker, 1994). On the other hand, if the view is that language is closely interrelated with other cognitive systems, then the idea of discrete linguistic difficulties would be untenable. The arguments surrounding the specific nature of language difficulties are somewhat similar to those surrounding dyslexia. Different camps have developed, with people taking extreme theoretical positions.

In practice the issue has revolved around how to define operationally a specific disorder of this type. This issue was first considered in Chapter 1. A rule of thumb has developed that a specific disorder is one that cannot be accounted for by other primary disorders such as low IQ, marked neurological difficulties, hearing impairment or primary emotional difficulties. It is also assumed that there are no significant adverse environmental factors that could explain the difficulties. Such a definition by exclusion has caused concern largely because it is unsatisfactory to define something by what it is not rather than what it is.

---

[2] Intervention refers to the allocation of additional services specifically directed at the needs of children with developmental language disorders.

In part the problem was one of clarity of the definitions adopted. This led Stark and Tallal in 1981 to place much closer constraints on what should be considered a specific problem. Since then a variety of different models of defining 'specific' have been adopted by different researchers and these have had a considerable impact on the way in which services have been provided in the US and the UK. In some cases services have only allowed children access to such services if they met the criterion concerned. The one feature that all these classificatory systems have in common is cognitive referencing: the definition of a specific discrepancy between language and performance IQ scores. Cognitive referencing makes it possible to be much more precise about the discrepancy. For example, authors quite often assume that one standard deviation (usually 15 points) on a standardized assessment is sufficient to warrant a diagnosis of specific language disorder. At one level such a discrepancy does make sense, and it is possible to show that such children do present with this profile (Conti-Ramsden et al., 1992). However, it is also statistically true that such discrepancies would be anticipated in the normal population and that they are not necessarily 'abnormal' (Cole et al., 1990; Aram et al., 1992). Indeed, such arguments have led some researchers in the field to suggest that the inappropriate application of standardized procedures can lead to disorders being created where they do not really exist (McFadden, 1996). This is not to say that there is no such thing as a language disorder, only that the concept tends to be extremely slippery when it comes to definition.

The issue of whether it is possible to define a discrete population also reflects on the extent to which it is possible to identify cases at an early stage in their development and effectively intervene to change the course of the disorder.

Identifying the need for specialist intervention in the early years

In the preschool period, speech and language therapists must make a judgement as to what, if any, specialist intervention is warranted and how it should best be provided. The thinking that makes up this judgement has to date remained somewhat opaque. It is assumed that the experience of the practitioner will allow him or her to digest the overall picture and come out with an appropriate solution. The result has been a 'black box' model of both diagnosis and intervention, which has proved rather resistant to replicable research. Some recent work on the diagnostic process has suggested that there is a degree of consensus both at the classificatory level and at the level of recommended action. For example, there have been a number of attempts to describe the way the experienced speech and language therapist reaches intervention decisions when assessing the preschool child. These have been both quantitative and qualitative in nature. For example Records and Tomblin (1994) looked at the way in which therapists interpreted test results and tried to ascertain where they started to determine that children had become cases. They concluded that case status did not follow the convention of –1 standard deviation but tended to be closer to –1.2 or near the tenth percentile. Roulstone by contrast adopted a qualitative methodology, using a notational tool known as 'systemic grammar networks' (Roulstone, 1997). This system allows the inclusion of all the relevant information that the speech and language therapist collects in judging whether a child needs specialist help, including historical aspects (family history, language and developmental history and both medical and environmental factors), the available options in terms of intervention – immediacy, length of session, and frequency, and the level of concern expressed by those closest to the child (parents, nursery staff, etc.).

It is of interest that the standardized assessment procedures in general and the discrepancy criterion in particular plays a very limited role in the description of the need for specialist help in the latter study. It seems likely that the priorities for practitioners are different from those of researchers, although it is to be hoped that there are links between the way the two groups construe clinical and educational issues. The practitioner by and large takes a strongly pragmatic line, reflecting on what evidence needs to be collected in order to do something, rather than describing exhaustively the condition in question.

For the professional to whom the child with a developmental language disorder is referred, some of the arguments related to the discrepancy between language and cognitive skills may appear somewhat arcane and, in practice, professionals often do not rely on discrepancy criteria. Rather they judge whether a child is adversely affected by the language difficulties that he or she experiences and whether there is an opportunity to intervene to modify a negative outcome. The differing perspectives of practitioners from different professional groups will be referred to in Chapter 5. Further, reliance on standardized procedures makes few allowances for the difficulties some children may experience in attending to test materials. This may be a function of a language impairment, but it may be a product simply of a limited attention span or an unfamiliarity with the materials of the assessment in question.

Whether intervention provided is significantly different for children with primary language disorders is somewhat unclear. There are clearly a great many features of intervention – such as optimizing the listening environment – which interventions have in common. Recently there has been considerable interest in psycholinguistic models of language processing as a framework for assessing such children and this probably does represent a discrete rationale which would be less likely to be employed with children with more general learning difficulties (Chiat et al., 1997; Stackhouse and Wells, 1997). The approach described in Chapter 4 is designed to have a broad application to language disorder across special needs groups.

Factors associated with developmental language disorder in the preschool period

Despite the general acceptance of the definition by exclusion, it has become apparent that even if it is not possible to account for their language difficulties in terms of other conditions, preschool children do present a complex picture. This includes a number of factors that may militate against the spontaneous resolution of difficulties even if they do not create the problem in the first place.

For example, there are a number of areas of cognitive development that are ostensibly normal but which are nevertheless lower than other skills. Symbolic development in general and play in particular are areas which have attracted considerable attention. There is a view that children with developmental language disorders may have impaired development of more general representational abilities (Leonard, 1987; Johnston, 1988; Tallal, 1988). Studies of language impaired children matched to language disordered children for age and for language level indicate that play lies somewhere between the lower language levels and the higher IQ (Kamhi, 1981). A review of studies into the symbolic play of language impaired children (Casby, 1997) indicates differences between receptive and expressive language disorders. Some studies have shown significant differences in the complexity of symbolic play between children with receptive language disorders and non-impaired groups (Udwin and Yule, 1983; Roth and Clark, 1987). However, studies by Lombardino et al. (1986) and Lovell et al. (1968) did not reveal significant differences in the complexity or amount of time spent in symbolic play activity between groups of children with expressive language disorders/delays and non-impaired children. The children with expressive disorders did show less complexity in their play activities at relatively older ages (4–5 years) but Casby (1997) suggests that here, the problem stems from language difficulty rather than a more general deficit in representational abilities. In particular, the children were less able to verbally comment or explicate their play schemas.

Equally, there is some suggestion that visual skills and numeracy may also be affected in children with specific language difficulties; not perhaps to the same extent as their language skills but nonetheless such that they are at a lower level than would be expected given other skills. In part this is an issue associated with the metrics that are now available to measure such skills. In the past such decisions were often made on the basis of professional judgement: more precise measurements mean more precise judgements but only if the risk of measurement error can be minimized. This is a particularly difficult issue when directly assessing the young child.

The issue of hearing loss is also one that bears consideration. Although it would be true to say that once children are found to have a sensorineural hearing loss they would be categorized separately, the same is not true for conductive hearing losses, particularly if they are intermittent as they are in many young children (Bishop and Edmundson, 1987b). Likewise, the issue of behavioural difficulties is one that has received considerable attention (Stevenson, 1996). It has long been observed that upwards of 50% of preschool children with language difficulties have behavioural difficulties as well (Cantwell and Baker, 1987). Such difficulties tend to be either of the externalizing acting out type or of the internalizing neurotic type and they tend to be more closely associated with language disorder than with speech disorder (Cantwell and Baker, 1987). It is widely accepted that they do not cause the language problems and it is commonly assumed that they are a function of it. Some authors have suggested that there is a neuro-developmental difficulty, which underlies both the language difficulty and the behaviour. It may be that associated temperamental presentations are what determines whether a child is likely to go on to have persistent language difficulties.

Attention deficits also frequently co-occur with language impairments. The child cannot communicate effectively and flits from one activity to another, never pausing long enough to make the connection between the objects to hand and their properties and the words that others in their environments use about them. Whether this is a behavioural 'problem' or a symptom of a broader neuro-developmental immaturity is often unclear.

The important point about these associated phenomena is that they may provide a key to measuring how likely it is that the child will have a persistent problem. They may therefore play as salient a role in identifying case status as a level of language delay measured on a standardized procedure, or the degree of discrepancy between language and other developmental skills.

What are the most important issues?

In order to meet the needs of children with developmental language difficulties it is necessary to go beyond the issues associated with classification. For the purposes of the present argument it is useful to examine four pieces of a jigsaw which, if they could be made to fit together, would represent a valuable approach to dealing with the identification and education/treatment of these children. To begin identifying the pieces of our jigsaw we need to start off with four questions:

- How large is the population of children with developmental language difficulties?
- Do they need to be identified, i.e. what happens to them when they do not receive intervention of any kind?
- What happens to them when they do receive intervention?
- How do we most effectively pick up those that need to be picked up – i.e. the ones whose difficulties do not resolve spontaneously?

These questions correspond to the four domains: **prevalence**, **natural history**, **intervention** and **screening**.

The literature from each area will be briefly summarized and a method will then be set out for examining the interrelationship between the four areas.

Prevalence up to 7 years

For many, prevalence occupies a central position in the analysis of developmental language disorders. Once prevalence can be established it will be possible to establish need and therefore make it possible to advocate the appropriate level of provision. Of course, it can work the other way around if prevalence is seen as representing the number of children whose condition would deteriorate significantly if they are not treated.

The prevalence literature related to children with developmental language disorders is complex because few studies appear to agree on how to categorize the cases concerned either in terms of the degree or the description of the disorder. In a recent systematic review of the literature in this area, the results from the best studies were summarized in terms of the median scores for speech difficulties alone, speech and language together and language difficulties alone. The findings are given in Table 2.1 (Law et al., 1998).

This synthesis excludes studies that did not use standardized procedures to identify prevalence. This makes for clearly replicable data and

Table 2.1 Median prevalence estimates by type of speech and language delay and age

Age	Type of impairment		
	Speech and language delay median percent [range]	Language delay only median percent [range]	Speech delay only median percent [range]
2;0 yr	5.0 [ ][a]	16 [8–19][b,]	–
3;0 yr	6.9 [5.6–8][a, c, d]	2.63 [0.6–7.6][e, f, g]	–
4;5 yr	5.0 [ ][a,]	–	–
5;0 yr	11.78 [4.56–19.0][h]	6.8 [2.14–10.4][f, h, i, j]	16.5 [6.4–24.6][h, i]
7;0 yr	–	3.1 [2.02–8.4][f]	2.3

Key [a] Bax et al. (1983) [b] Rescorla et al. (1993) [c] Burden et al. (1996) [d] Randall et al. (1974) [e] Stevenson and Richman (1976) [f] Silva et al. (1983) [g] Wong et al. (1992) [h] Beitchman et al. (1986) [i] Tuomi and Ivanoff (1977) [j] Tomblin et al. (1997) .

cuts out much of the wide variation that tends to occur when specialists are asked to make judgements about whether a child is experiencing a difficulty. When such judgements are made it is impossible not to reject the possibility that prevalence is more a function of the level of resources than an absolute level of difficulty. The more specialists and services available to meet the needs of such children, the higher the prevalence. The negative side of using standardized procedures as a means of ascertaining whether children are experiencing difficulties is that the data tend to become circular: researchers set their cut-offs on the standardized procedures according to the level they consider to represent a problem. They then find that the prevalence data reflect that level and any discrepancy between the predicted prevalence and the identified prevalence is more a function of the difference between the population under investigation and the population upon whom the test in question was originally standardized.

The other area of difference is the level at which measures are set. The range reported was 0.6% to 24.6%, suggesting that practitioners and researchers have very different perceptions of what needs to be identified. Of course, prevalence levels in themselves do not necessarily presuppose that the authors are assuming that all the children identified should receive specialist help. Indeed, with the exception of one or two studies, no clinical or educational rationale is given for the levels set. This is an oversight, and one that needs to be addressed if developmental language disorders are to be a meaningful construct. Until the clinical status of the children identified is clarified it will not be possible to make any meaningful estimates of need.

Natural history

Natural history refers to what happens to the children identified when they do not receive intervention. If we can answer this then it should be possible to target the children at greatest risk for persistent problems. This is a somewhat difficult concept to address in this field for a number of reasons:

1) Children do not receive nothing if they do not receive specialist help. They are usually in regular contact with adults who are able to provide a 'good enough' environment. Of course there are cases of children raised in isolation, but these are extreme examples and probably do not help this argument very much (Skuse, 1988). This raises the question of what it means to have a 'natural' history.
2) In societies where there are existing services in place to help such children it is probably difficult to withhold such services for any length of time for the purposes of empirical investigation.
3) Life events and experiences may intervene to interfere with the child's orientation to learning. This may depress tested language scores. So an individual child's performance may deteriorate as well as improve.
4) It is not easy to provide continuous data sets on a single metric throughout the course of a study because language measures often do not span the desired age range. In practice, researchers often replace language measures with measures of reading, IQ, etc.
5) The language measures used may give the impression of children crossing a line between normality and case status. This may be a real change but it may also be a function of the test–retest reliability of the measure itself.
6) Performance on a test does not necessarily reflect whether a child has a problem. This is a somewhat unclear issue and it might be reasonable to argue that the testing procedure may over-identify, especially in the first few years of life when development is extremely noisy and when children may respond poorly to the unfamiliar nature of the testing situation. It seems relatively unlikely that children who perform reasonably well on formal procedures will be manifesting a covert problem. There are exceptions to this, in the area of pragmatic impairments in particular, and these will be referred to in Chapter 3.

Nonetheless, from the data that are available it is possible to say there appears to be a relatively high rate of spontaneous recovery across the age span. This recovery rate tends to decline with age and is also sensitive to a number of 'within child' measures. So between 2 and 3 years from 40 to 65% of children with expressive delays have problems which resolve spontaneously. Thereafter the picture becomes less clear. Fiedler et al. (1971) suggest that this figure decreases still further to 38% if the range is increased (2–7 years). The benchmark study that has contributed most to our understanding of natural history in this area is that from Dunedin, New Zealand (Silva et al., 1983). In this study it is possible to trace children from 3 to 11 years. Between 3 and 5 years the researcher found 30/37 (81%) to have continual problems; between 5 and 7 years there were 25/48 (52%) who continued to have problems and between 3 and 7 the figures were 23/39 (58%). Even these figures give a slightly misleading impression of the continuity, however, because it is apparent that children were moving out of the problem group and back in again. Of the original 37 cases, only 17 (46%) had problems throughout the study.

If these results are contrasted with the history of a group for whom intervention was provided but at an unquantifiable level a rather different picture emerges. The best example is the cohort identified by Bishop and Edmundson (1987a) when the children were 4, and followed through to 15 years (Stothard et al., 1998). Of the 71 children that the researchers were able to follow up, 15 had originally been diagnosed as having more general difficulties while 56 had specific language impairment. By 5;6 months 26 of those 56 (46%) had problems which had resolved. Of the remaining 30, 21 (70%) continued to have specific language impairment nearly ten years later and a further 6 (20%) now had more general learning difficulties. So by 5;6 it was possible to predict future case status with 90% accuracy.

The story that emerges here is that the earlier children are identified, the more difficult it is to predict whether they really are going to experience problems later on. This is particularly true for children with expressive language delays. There is a need for a process for more accurately predicting subsequent performance in the early years. The evidence here suggests that expressive language performance in its own right is not sufficient. Adding receptive language to the equation makes a considerable difference. Nevertheless, one could argue that any sign of potential delay would be cause enough for intervention to be recommended. This would mean that all the appropriate children would receive intervention, but a large sample of children who do not need specialist help would also be seen. This is not a trivial matter. Apart from the costs to the service providers, it is very likely that there will be costs to individuals who receive specialist help when they don't need it. These may be in terms of psychological costs to the individual child and in terms of lowered expectations on the part of parents and teachers. To a certain extent this may be avoided in an educational context where it may be easier not to stigmatize children through the identification process.

Intervention

Intervention refers to the allocation of additional services specifically directed at the needs of the children with developmental language impairment. A great many adults from the parents to the nursery teacher will provide input throughout the preschool years. There are many such interventions and it is impossible to say whether they are all equally valid. However, a picture is now emerging from the literature of the positive impact of a range of interventions. The interested reader is referred to McClean and Woods Cripe (1997) for a narrative account and Law et al. (1998) for a syntheses of effect sizes across studies. Indeed, McClean and Woods Cripe argue that we should be moving away from first-order research – establishing whether intervention works or not – and start to look for differential impacts of different interventions on different individuals. The conclusion from Law et al. is rather more cautious because it suggests that there is strong evidence of effects in certain areas, most notably expressive delays, but much less evidence for the group identified as being most at risk for persistent delays: notably children with receptive language delays. The data support the finding that indirect intervention, notably through parents, can be as effective as direct intervention and suggest that it is difficult to differentiate between the effects of different types of intervention at this stage.

In the discussion to date the assumption has effectively been made that intervention in the preschool period comprises specialist provision made by speech and language therapists in isolation from other services. While this is certainly very relevant it does not represent the complete picture. Although nursery services in the UK are currently underdeveloped relative to other countries in the EU, the fact is that by 4 years of age many of these children will have experienced some sort of nursery provision. Evaluation of intervention provided in such circumstances has not been well described. Most of the emphasis has been on developing and providing programmes for nursery staff to use. One notable exception to this is Best et al.'s examination of an intervention programme in a social services day nursery (Best et al., 1993). This aspect of indirect work is one that will need further investigation in future. If the impact on significant others is as potent as it seems to be on parents, such intervention will be construed as a valuable alternative to conventional health clinic focused services. However, given recent evidence on the nature of daycare and nursery services there is good reason to be cautious in assuming that intervention in such circumstances will provide a panacea unless sufficient resources are made available for the individual concerned (Melhuish and Moss, 1990). The consultant role of the speech and language therapist in optimizing the input for all children with developmental language disorders is one which will also deserve close scrutiny in the future.

It is often argued that the real test of whether intervention can be said to work is not the experience of the individual child or family; not the effect of a particular educational programme, but evidence of declining prevalence in the population as a whole. The prevalence data reported above do not allow for such a judgement because they are too disparate and reflect too diverse a range of different service providers in a number of different countries. Only one study has explicitly referred to the provision of intervention services as a possible explanation of a declining prevalence (Bax et al., 1983). In this study prevalence of definitely abnormal cases between 2 years, 3 years and 4;6 years rose slightly and then fell from 5% to 8% and back to 5% but during the same period the number of possibly abnormal cases fell consistently from 17% to 12% to 7%. The effects of intervention at this level are only speculative at this stage. Nonetheless, the picture that emerges regarding intervention for expressive language delays is a positive one.

The nature of intervention in the preschool period, in particular, in relation to needs at school entry, is further discussed in Chapter 4.

Screening

Within the NHS in the UK there is a general acceptance of the need to provide developmental surveillance, identifying children in need of help because they are visually impaired or if a child's development is generally delayed. Although there is some uncertainty about the precise meaning of the concept 'developmental surveillance', with regard to speech and language development it is generally understood to be a screening programme whereby primary healthcare professionals use their judgement or some sort of measure to ascertain whether a given child needs to be referred for further assessment by a speech and language therapist or by the team in a child development centre.

Screening programmes for children were originally introduced for circumscribed medical conditions such as phenylketonuria, and although attempts have been made to apply the same criteria for variables which follow a Gaussian distribution – i.e. are normally distributed – they have left many with a sense of scepticism as to whether behaviour and language can ever be divided into 'normal' and 'abnormal' in any satisfactory way. Nonetheless, such measures do exist and are relatively widely used.

The main criteria for their success is the extent to which they accurately distinguish children who really are cases from those who are not, while not missing cases within the normal population. The terms used to describe the accuracy are *sensitivity* and *specificity* respectively. A sensitive measure is one that misses very few children; a specific measure is one that does not over-identify children. Conventionally acceptable levels of specificity and sensitivity are said to be in the region of 0.8. In the review of the literature referred to above (Law et al., 1998) it was clear that the majority of measures do in fact meet these criteria. Does screening therefore work? Within its own terms the answer to this would seem to be yes. However, on closer inspection the answer is rather more complicated. As part of the evaluation of any screening procedure it is necessary to determine before the evaluation the level at which a case becomes a case, in other words what cut-off should be adopted. This applies to the gold standard measure and also to the screening test itself. Table 2.2 indicates the range of cut-offs adopted for the various screening tests.

Table 2.2 Variety of cut-off score definitions for reference tests

By chronological age (CA)/language age	By standard deviations	By standard scores	By centile scores	Other
–6 months –12 months	–1 –1.5	Less than 80 Less than 85	Less than 10th, 15th, 25th, 30th centile	Language sample analysis
	–2			at stage III
Less than two-thirds of CA				3 subtests failed of a test
Less than 0.7 of CA				'Severe' score

Irrespective of whether a formal screening test is adopted the problem will remain the same until we have some understanding of the pre-test probability of an individual becoming a case. We will not be able to say whether a screening test can pick up an objectively definable case. It is for this reason that in the following section the interrelationships between the key areas of concern are drawn out for those studying developmentally language disordered children.

In Figure 2.1 the different parts of the developmental language disorder jigsaw are drawn together. It shows how the areas are interrelated: something that has received scant attention in the literature to date. A case of developmental language disorder is one that stands to benefit from intervention and will not otherwise resolve. Whether it is possible to identify cases consistently across a population depends upon there being a measure that can be applied universally by primary care workers and is supported by the necessary predictive evidence. Such a model takes the emphasis away from the often rather stale discussions of classification.

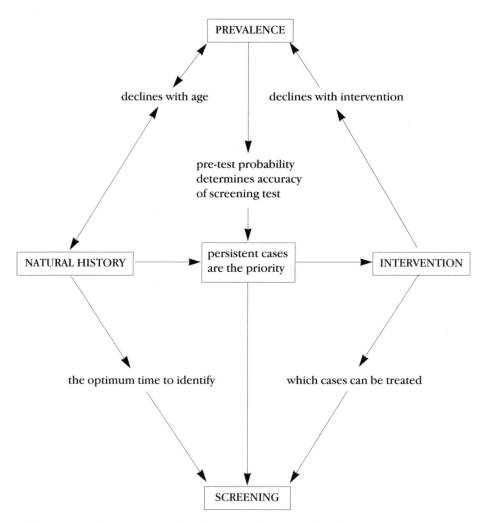

Figure 2.1 A dynamic view of developmental language disorder.

Conclusion

The conclusion drawn from our systematic review in this area was that there was insufficient evidence at this stage to warrant universal screening for speech and language impairment because there are too many gaps in the literature to have confidence in the authority of such a process (Law et al., 1998). But these conclusions refer only to screening. There is now a mass of evidence to suggest the benefits of intervention, and it should be this evidence that drives the identification and classification process in the future.

It needs to be recognized that children with specific developmental language disorders, while their difficulties may be construed as primarily pertaining to language, also experience a wide range of other problems. If such children are to be provided with a comprehensive service, both the categorization and definitions of such disorders need to take this into consideration. One of the weaknesses of the review referred to above is that outcomes were confined to those relating to speech and language. In future the impact of intervention, and indeed outcomes of natural history studies, will need to reflect this broadening of the way that language disorders are conceptualized and, most notably, how they impact on the educational process.

Having demonstrated that there is value in the process of intervention, there is a case for developing a greater understanding of that process and for identifying a) how diagnostic decisions are made and b) how the intervention is carried out with regard to the individual child. The nature of specialist or therapeutic interventions is that they reflect an interactive process between practitioner and individual, the subtleties of which will be overshadowed in the sometimes rather clumsy process of efficacy evaluation. This should then help us address the issue of how some children stand to benefit from intervention and some do not. It will also help us address the issue of whether we are trying to remove the disorder, or to lessen its impact.

References

Adams C, Byers-Brown B, Edwards M. Developmental Disorders of Language (2nd edition). London: Whurr Publishers Ltd, 1997.

Aram D, Morris R, Hall N. The validity of discrepancy criteria for identifying children with developmental language disorders. Journal of Learning Disabilities 1992; 25 (9): 549–54.

Bax M, Hart H, Jenkins S. The behaviour, development and health of the young child: implications for care. British Medical Journal 1983; 286: 1793–6.

Beitchman JH, Nair R, Clegg M, Patel PG, Ferguson B, Pressman E, et al. Prevalence of speech and language disorders in 5-year-old kindergarten children in the Ottawa-Carleton region. Journal of Speech and Hearing Disorders 1986; 51(2): 98–110.

Best W, Melvin D, Williams S. The effectiveness of communication groups in day nurseries. European Journal of Disorders of Communication 1993; 28 (2): 187–212.

Bishop DVM. The underlying nature of specific language impairment. Journal of Child Psychology and Psychiatry 1992; 33 (1): 3–66.

Bishop DVM, Edmundson A. Language impaired 4 year olds: distinguishing transient from persistent impairment. Journal of Speech and Hearing Disorders 1987[a]; 52: 156–73.

Bishop DVM, Edmundson A. Is otitis media a major cause of specific developmental language disorders? British Journal of Disorders of Communication 1987[b]; 21: 321–38.

Burden V, Stott CM, Forge J, Goodyer I. The Cambridge Language and Speech Project (CLASP). 1. Detection of language difficulties at 36–39 months. Developmental Medicine and Child Neurology 1996; 38 (7): 613–31.

Cantwell DP, Baker L. Prevalence and types of psychiatric disorders in three speech and language groups. Journal of Communication Disorders 1987; 20: 151–60.

Casby MW. Symbolic play of children with language impairment: a critical review. Journal of Speech and Hearing Research 1997; 40: 468–79.

Chiat S, Law J, Marshall J. Language Disorders in Children and Adults: Psycholinguistic Approaches to Therapy. London: Whurr Publishers Ltd, 1997.

Cole P, Dale K, Mills P. Defining language delay in young children by cognitive referencing: are we saying more than we know? Applied Psycholinguistics 1990; 11: 291–302.

Conti-Ramsden G, Donlan C, Grove J. Characteristics of children with specific language impairment attending language units. European Journal of Disorders of Communication 1992; 27 (4): 325–43.

Fiedler MF, Lenneberg EH, Rolfe UT, Droorbaugh JE. A speech screening procedure with three-year-old children. Pediatrics 1971; 48 (2): 268–76.

Johnston. Specific language disorders in the child. In Lass N, McReynolds L, Northern J, Yoder D (eds) Handbook of Speech-language Pathology and Audiology. Toronto: BC Decker, 1988.

Kamhi A. Non linguistic symbolic and conceptual abilities of language impaired and normally developing children. Journal of Speech and Hearing Research 1981; 24: 446–53.

Law J. Evaluating early intervention for language impaired children: a review of the literature. European Journal of Disorders of Communication 1997; 32: 1–14.

Law J, Boyle J, Harris F, Harkness A. Screening for speech and language delay: a systematic review of the literature. Health Technology Assessment 1998; 2 (9).

Leonard L. Is specific language impairment a useful construct? In Rosenberg S (ed) Advances in Applied Psycholinguistics, Volume 1. Chichester: Lawrence Erlbaum, 1987.

Lombardino L, Stein J, Kricos P, Wolf M. Play diversity and structural relationships in the play and language of language-impaired and language-normal preschoolers. Preliminary data. Journal of Communication Disorders 1986; 19: 475–89.

Lovell K, Hoyle H, Sidall M. A study of some aspects of the play and language of young children with delayed speech. Journal of Child Psychology and Psychiatry 1968; 9: 41–50.

McClean LK, Woods Cripe JW. The effectiveness of early intervention for children with communication disorders. In Guralnick MJ (ed) The Effectiveness of Early Intervention. Baltimore, MD: Paul H. Brookes, 1997.

McFadden T. Creating language impairment in typically achieving children: the pitfalls of 'normal' normative sampling. Language Speech and Hearing Services in Schools 1996; 27: 3–9.

Melhuish EC, Moss P (eds). Day Care for Young Children: International Perspectives. London: Routledge, 1990.

Pinker S. The Language Instinct: The New Science of Language and Mind. London: The Penguin Press, 1994.

Randall D, Reynell J, Curwen M. A study of language development in a sample of 3 year old children. British Journal of Disorders of Communication 1974; 9 (1): 3–16.

Records NL, Tomblin JB. Clinical decision making: describing the decision rules of practising speech-language pathologists. Journal of Speech and Language Research 1994; 37: 144–56.

Rescorla L, Hadicke-Wiley M, Escarce E. Epidemiological investigation of expressive language delay at age two. Special Issue: Language development in special populations. First Language 1993; 13 (37, Pt 1): 5–22.

Roth F, Clark D. Symbolic play and social participation abilities of language impaired and normally developing children. Journal of Speech and Hearing Research 1987; 52: 17–29.

Roulstone S. What's driving you? A template which underpins the assessment of pre-school children by speech and language therapists. European Journal of Disorders in Human Communication 1997; 32 (3): 299–317.

Silva PA, McGee R, Williams SM. Developmental language delay from three to seven years and its significance for low intelligence and reading difficulties at age seven. Developmental Medicine and Child Neurology 1983; 25: 783–93.

Skuse D. Extreme deprivation in early childhood. In Bishop DVM, Mogford K (eds) Language Development in Exceptional Circumstances. Edinburgh: Churchill Livingstone, 1988, pp. 29–46.

Stackhouse J, Wells B. Children's Speech and Literacy Difficulties: A Psycholinguistic Framework. London: Whurr Publishers Ltd, 1997.

Stark R, Tallal P. Selection of children with specific language deficits. Journal of Speech and Hearing Disorders 1981; 46: 114–22.

Stevenson J. Developmental changes in the mechanism linking language disabilities and behavior disorders. In Beitchman J, Cohen N, Konstantareas MM, Tannock R (eds) Language Learning and Behavior Disorders: Developmental, Biological and Clinical Perspectives. Cambridge: Cambridge University Press, 1996.

Stevenson J, Richman N. The prevalence of language delay in a population of three-year-old children and its association with general retardation. Developmental Medicine and Child Neurology 1976; 18 (4): 431–41.

Stothard SE, Snowling MJ, Bishop DVM, Chipchase BB, Kaplan CA. Language impaired pre-schoolers: a follow-up into adolescence. Journal of Speech, Language and Hearing Disorders 1998; 41: 407–18.

Tallal P. Developmental language disorders. In Kavanagh J, Truss T Jr (eds) Learning Disabilities: Proceedings of the National Conference. Parkton, MD: New York Press, 1988.

Tallal P, Merzenich MM, Miller S, Jenkins A. Language learning impairments: integrating basic science, technology and remediation. Experimental Brain Research 1998; 123: 210–19.

Terrel BY, Schwartz RG, Prelock PA, Messick CK. Symbolic play in normal and language impaired children. Journal of Speech and Hearing Research 1984; 27: 424–9.

Tomblin JB, Records N, Buckwalter P, Zhang X, Smith E, O'Brien M. Prevalence of specific language impairment in kindergarten children. Journal of Speech Language and Hearing Research 1997; 40 (6): 1245–60.

Tuomi S, Ivanoff P. Incidence of speech and hearing disorders among kindergarten and grade 1 children. Special Education in Canada 1977; 51 (4): 5–8.

Udwin O, Yule W. Imaginative play in language disordered children. British Journal of Disorders of Communication 1983; 18 (3): 197–205.

Wong V, Lee PWH, Mak-Lieh F, Yeung CY, Leung PWL, Luk SL, et al. Language screening in pre-school Chinese children. European Journal of Disorders of Communication 1992; 27 (3): 247–64.

Chapter 3
A pragmatic disorder in the contexts of autism and developmental language disorder

WENDY RINALDI

Introduction

A great deal of interest and debate surrounds a group of children who traditionally were viewed in the *language disorder* category, as 'semantic–pragmatic syndrome' (Rapin and Allen, 1987) (renamed semantic–pragmatic disorder; Bishop and Adams, 1989), but who would be more accurately described *autistic* according to some (Brook and Bowler, 1992, 1998; Aarons and Gittens, 1998; Happe, 1994). It will be proposed in this chapter that a more accurate description of this condition is a *pragmatic disorder* and that a fuller understanding of this disorder will provide a key to how these children can most helpfully be considered in terms of intervention and educational placement. The chapter will then examine the case for pragmatic disorder in the context of developmental language disorder and in the context of autism.

What is a pragmatic disorder?

The first step is to attempt to get to grips with the notion of a pragmatic disorder, since this can be viewed as a key to understanding and developing children's knowledge and skills, regardless of the diagnostic category applied: autism/autism spectrum disorder, semantic–pragmatic disorder, Asperger's syndrome, pervasive developmental disorder. This is important because currently the diagnostic label applied can depend on which professional the child has seen (Bishop, 1989). That is, whichever label is used, the children's difficulties include a pragmatic disorder, usually to a significant degree. The author makes this claim based on her experience of many children referred under the gamut of labels outlined above.

41

So what is a pragmatic disorder? The definitions of pragmatics outlined in Figure 3.1 are drawn from a literature review scanning the last 50 years or so.

- Morris (1938) Semantics: the relation of signs to the objects to which they are applicable
  Pragmatics: the relation of signs to **interpreters**

- Bloom and Lahey (1978)
  - Content (semantics): the topics that are represented in messages (a topic being an idea such as a reference to an object, action or relation)
  - Use (pragmatics): the influence of **linguistic and non-linguistic context** on how individuals understand and **choose** among alternative forms of language

- Levinson (1983) Pragmatics = meaning minus semantics

- Leech (1983) Semantics: meaning as a dyadic relation, as in 'what does X mean?'
  Pragmatics: meaning in a **triadic** relation, as in 'what did you mean by X?'

- Roth and Spekman (1984) Pragmatics is at the **interface of social, cognitive and linguistic knowledge**

- Crystal (1987) Pragmatics: '**assumptions** that people make when they communicate, the **intentions** underlying what they say, the way **context influences** the amount they say or the way they say it, the **turn-taking** which makes a conversation run smoothly and the **appropriateness** of the subject matter to the situation'

Figure 3.1 Definitions of pragmatics and semantics.

Crystal's definition provides perhaps the most comprehensive overview, but it does emphasize language use/expression. Indeed, the consideration of pragmatics exclusively within the domain of language use, as suggested by Bloom and Lahey's model of language, is potentially misleading because, as made clear by many other definitions, there is an area of pragmatics that concerns comprehension. The following three aspects of communication summarize the areas of pragmatics mentioned in the definitions and provide a mechanism for understanding the ways in which pragmatics may be disrupted.

- The interactive process of communication
- The selection and organization of information/ideas within the communicative context
- The comprehension of meaning open to interpretation

Children with pragmatic disorders show significant difficulty with these aspects of communication in relation to other aspects of the language profile (for example, phonology, grammar, word knowledge/word-finding abilities), as illustrated in the following sections.

The interactive process of communication

There are a number of ways in which the interactive process of communication may be disrupted. Children may, for example, show difficulty in one or more of the following:

- Initiating communication. Difficulties here may arise because the child fails to use non-verbal signals (such as eye contact, body posture, proximity) to show a desire to communicate.
- 'Handing over' the speaker role/allowing the listener to respond. Children can appear to dominate conversations because of low awareness of the speaker–listener exchange, in particular the need to 'share' the speaker role with conversational partners.
- Timing of turns. Mistiming conversational turns causes children to interrupt the speaker and gives the impression of poor listening/low interest in others' talk.
- 'Conversational repairs' describe attempts by speakers and listeners to resolve factors that could cause a breakdown in communication. One instance of conversational repair, which in particular involves the interactive process of communication, concerns how speakers manage a situation when they initiate a communication at the same time. When this occurs, a conversation can be 'repaired' by one of the speakers suspending their turn to allow the other speaker to continue, taking up their turn at a later stage in the conversation. Children who fail to repair conversations will continue to speak in parallel.

Teaching/therapy can develop children's awareness of speaker/listener roles and the strategies/skills needed in switching between them (Rustin and Kuhr, 1989; Rinaldi, 1992, 1995, 1996; Kelly, 1996).

Selection and organization of information/ideas according to listener need

There are a number of features that indicate a difficulty with language selection and organizational abilities. In the main, these concern three overlapping areas: sufficiency, relevance and coherence.

Difficulties with language selection and organization show themselves most clearly when children attempt to communicate from a start point that requires them to make choices from a range of possibilities. Examples include: describing/explaining an event, telling or writing a story, answering 'open' questions (such as *Tell me about your family*). In these instances the content is familiar, but it is the decision as to which information to include which poses the difficulty: What does the listener need to know? What will interest them? How much information should be given in the time available? When the listener cues the child or asks less open questions (such as *Who is in your family?/ Where do you live?*), the number of choices required is reduced and the difficulty becomes less evident.

Teaching/ therapy can be focused to enable children to self-cue, to develop a greater awareness of the needs of listeners and to develop strategies for selection and planning that will enable them to make more effective language choices (Rinaldi, 1999).

These considerations can be located in the pragmatic area because decisions about listener need (and the effects of listener cueing) occur only within the context of the communication process. It is clear that semantic (linguistic and cognitive) skills and strategies enable more effective language organization, particularly in the area of cohesion, as will be described later in this section. However, it is quite possible that a semantic analysis of a child's expression will not reveal problems with communicative relevance or coherence, when a problem does in fact exist. For example, vocabulary and semantic relations may be appropriately expressed. There may be a logical sequence to irrelevant information: a child may become extremely detailed about a particular aspect of content without covering more general information needed to enable the listener to follow. Outside the communicative context, a semantic analysis would not reveal any difficulty here.

Distinctions between semantics and pragmatics are covered in more depth later in this chapter.

The following sections illustrate the effects of difficulties with sufficiency, relevance and coherence.

Sufficiency

Children may have such difficulty in selecting appropriate information that either they are not able to formulate a response (they may say 'don't know'), or they respond in a very limited way. When the listener provides cues or less open questions this reveals that the child does in fact know the information: it was the difficulty in selecting from the array of alternatives that prevented the child from responding.

Figure 3.2 illustrates this kind of difficulty with four examples. In the first two examples, the children are able to verbalize the difficulty. In examples 2 and 4 the children are not only aware of the difficulty but also are aware of a strategy that will assist them; that is, to invite the listener to ask them further questions.

Example 1

Therapist: *Tell me about your family.*

Child (CA 12;10): '*I have – there's lots of them ... I can't ... there's ... oh ...' (child signals frustration)*

Example 2

Therapist: *Tell me about yourself.*

Child (CA 13;02): '*Oh mmm, no I can't ... like what? What do you want to know about me?'*

Example 3

Therapist: *What's your room like?*

Child (CA 11;8): '*Well it's big – yeah quite big. Got my computer in there and the bunks – two bunks – and it's got brown in there and flowers.'*

Therapist: *Got brown in there?*

Child: *Yeah on the flowers – and my toys are in there ...*

Example 4

Therapist: *Tell me about yourself. Have a think and tell me everything you can.*

Child (CA 12;06): '*Eh? (long pause) it's not like we're writing letters, so why don't you ask me questions. Curiosity is stronger than thinking about things – you've got the curiosity whereas I'm just thinking of things.'*

Figure 3.2 Examples to illustrate difficulties in language selection.

A further feature that can affect sufficiency (and coherence) is the ability to mark reference adequately. This kind of difficulty is illustrated in example 3: the listener is unable to make sense of 'got brown in there' because the child has not made it clear what this description refers to. Another example of a difficulty with reference-marking, often seen in children with pragmatic difficulties, concerns nominal reference; that is the appropriate use of nouns and pronouns. In particular, the child may a) refer to names of people, places, animals, objects (e.g. toys) without referring to whom or what they are (an example of this is asterisked in example 2 of Figure 3.3) or b) over-use pronouns without making reference to the associated nouns: that is, the child refers to 'he', 'she', 'it' 'we', etc., without naming the people or objects referred to.

Relevance

Figure 3.3 includes examples of difficulty in selecting relevant informa-tion. In example 1, the child fails to mention that he is describing a cup; the listener is therefore unable to form an accurate mental picture. The child also omits important information such as object function. In example 2, the child gives a lot of detail about a particular event, but this is not the information sought by the question posed.

Example 1[1]

Therapist: *So tell me about the thing you've taken out the bag.*

Child (CA 11;05): 'Well, it's plastic. There are circles at the bottom and a black dot. (The child is describing circular grooves in the plastic at the base of the cup and a speck of dirt.) There are flowers on the outside.'

Example 2

Therapist: *Tell me about yourself. Have a think and tell me everything you can.*

Child (CA 9;07): 'I'm a child who lives in —— (names town) I live with my mum and dad in all the parts of —— (names county). Early Monday mornings I get up and go to school – I sometimes go with mum or dad. We got up at seven, I tried to be early but he* wouldn't listen. I have a snack – it's just my motorway snack – and I have a carton drink too. I am at ——-school (names school).'

Figure 3.3 Examples to illustrate a difficulty with relevance.

Coherence

Language is usually organized to incorporate the following features:

- An overview or introduction to a theme or theme shift: for example, *we got back from our holiday yesterday*; *I must tell you about next weekend*. This is sometimes referred to as 'signposting'.
- Within each theme, a selection of topics or categories linked by some logical sequence. For example, *we got back from holiday yesterday* (theme): *the weather was fantastic – sun every day – it only rained once (topic 1: weather)......*[2] *we spent a lot of time sunbathing but I managed to get in some sightseeing – the Taj Mahal was out of this world* (topic 2: what did) *....... but I must tell you about next weekend* (theme shift).

---

[1] In this activity, the therapist gives the child a bag of objects. The instructions to the child are that they must tell everything about the object so that the therapist can make a picture of it. The therapist does not see the object whilst the child is describing it.
[2] ... indicates time allowed for the listener's response.

The ability to formulate coherent communication depends upon the ability to 'chunk' information into themes and themes into topics. This skill is assisted by an awareness of categorization. Experience has shown that attaching a verbal label to information (e.g. holiday, weekend, etc.) assists in the 'chunking' process. A sense of hierarchical planning also assists in this process, in particular, considering the relation between categories applied to themes and topics. For example:

HOLIDAY → **weather** → sun, rain once
　　　　　　　 → **what did** → sunbathe, sightseeing → Taj Mahal

NEXT WEEKEND →

Difficulties with coherence can result in the child's talk having a rambling quality because there is no obvious logical sequence to their ideas, as illustrated in the example in Figure 3.4

Therapist: *Tell me about your family.*

Child (CA 12;09): Well my mum works in a hairdressers and she goes to this shop place. I got *Rangers Go Wild* I did. My dad took me at the weekend. Yeah and we live at—(recites address). So, but you can't go in on Sundays. Mum tried to get in there 'cause she left her purse behind. Yeah, Mark hit me he did – I got a bruise – look.

Figure 3.4 Example of a difficulty with coherence.

Another form of difficulty occurs when the child includes one theme only, developing it into minute detail of less interest to the listener. There is clearly also a problem of relevance here, as illustrated in Figure 3.3, example 2.

Comprehension of meaning open to interpretation

In Figure 3.1, definitions by Leech, Morris, and Bloom and Lahey in particular highlighted the difference between semantic and pragmatic comprehension. In semantic comprehension, the meaning conveyed is in terms of a direct correspondence between idea (for example, object, event, relation) and form (for example, word, phrase, sentence). Difficulties in this area are demonstrated by, for example, gaps in vocabulary, conceptual or morphological[3] knowledge.

Pragmatic comprehension concerns meaning open to interpretation and requires the listener to make a choice about the speaker's intended

---

[3] A morpheme is a minimum meaning bearing unit, including grammatical markers. For example, plural /s/ means *more than one.*

meaning. It is an appreciation of **contextual understanding** which enables resolution of the ambiguity. Lexically, the word 'semantics' is equated with meaning; however, there is justification for considering the resolution of ambiguous meaning apart from semantics because the resolution of ambiguity may be governed by factors not concerning semantics. As identified by Bloom and Lahey (1978), context can sometimes even fall outside the domain of language but, here, the consideration of pragmatics is how non-linguistic information can impinge upon language meaning. The following three examples illustrate the types of contextual information that children may need to consider to comprehend meaning open to interpretation.

Example 1. **Homonym: jam (meaning 1: sweet conserve; meaning 2: an obstruction/block)**

Situational context: A staff meeting is under way; a teacher enters the room and says:

'I'm sorry I'm late, the motorway was completely jammed'

Linguistic context: Semantically, the word 'motorway' indicates a traffic jam. The notion of a road being covered in (strawberry) jam is implausible. Grammatically, only the second meaning can be expressed in verb form.

Example 2. **Pull socks up (meaning 1: literal; meaning 2: idiomatic)**

Situational context: A teacher is handing back Maths homework. Jenny has got most of it wrong (she isn't wearing socks). The teacher says:

'Jenny, if you want to pass your GCSE you'll have to pull your socks up'

Linguistic context: Semantically, the need to pass an exam would infer an idiomatic meaning.

It should be noted that the knowledge of multiple or idiomatic meanings per se concerns semantics; however it is the **choice** of speaker intention (and the need to determine choice according to plausibility, grammatical congruity, etc.) that concerns the area of pragmatics.

Research into how non-impaired children understand new idiomatic or multiple meanings sheds some light on the processes that may be involved as children develop pragmatic comprehension. There is evidence in the literature that children first acquire an understanding of idioms through familiarity (Ackerman, 1982; Cacciari and Levorato, 1989); that is, as a result of people explaining different meanings to them. There is also some evidence that young primary school children (6–8 years) have some sense of plausibility, but do not seek alternatives to literal meanings (Rinaldi, 2000). At 10+ years children are able to rule out meanings rendered implausible by context. If they don't know the implied or idiomatic meaning they will make an informed guess, based on the context, or assert that they don't know (Cacciari and Levorato, 1989; Rinaldi, 2000).

Children with pragmatic disorders have particular difficulty with these kinds of processes. Although they may have the semantic knowledge needed to interpret idiomatic and multiple meanings and may be able to do well when items are presented out of context, they are unable to complete the necessary pragmatic processing to comprehend speaker intention. The studies cited in the previous paragraph indicate that this processing includes plausibility judgement, awareness of the need to seek alternative referents and the ability to detect miscomprehension. Rinaldi (2000) proposes a model to account for the different ways in which these processes may break down at a metacommunicative level (awareness of the need to perform pragmatic analyses) and/or at a language level.

A pragmatic approach to teaching/therapy is to focus children's awareness on the need to consider context in interpreting multiple meanings and to develop strategies for comprehension monitoring (Rinaldi, 1996a).

Example 3. **Inconsistency between verbal and non-verbal communication**

Situational context: A family has been out shopping – the back seat of their car is loaded with shopping bags. Parent says to child:

'Oh dear! Looks like there's no room for you – we'll have to leave you here!'

Non-verbal context: parent smiles. Tone of voice indicates they are joking – they don't mean what they are saying.

Here, the situational context does not serve to resolve the ambiguity. It is the non-verbal communication that indicates the speaker's intended meaning: that is, that they are joking and aren't going to leave the child behind.

This kind of ambiguity is different from the previous two examples in that the speaker deliberately makes the communication ambiguous, intending the listener to note the inconsistency and realize that they are joking. This kind of communication was referred to in Grice's (1975) cooperative principle, which identifies that sometimes speakers deliberately flout rules of cooperation in communication (one such rule is to be clear and unambiguous) to add to meaning.

In this example the verbal *and* non-verbal message can be located within the domain of semantics. In both message types the speaker is expressing ideas, but is using different signals to express them (words; facial expression and tone of voice). However it is the appreciation of the manipulation of communication and the choice of which message carries speaker intention that concerns pragmatic comprehension. The speaker may assume the listener will realize that ambiguity contributes to the meaning of the communication, but children with a pragmatic disorder may not know how to interpret such inconsistency even in those cases where they are able to detect it (Rinaldi, 2000).

A pragmatic approach to teaching/therapy focuses upon developing an awareness of inconsistency and how to interpret it (Rinaldi, 1996).

Cognitive and social abilities of children with a pragmatic disorder

The nature of pragmatics at the interface of linguistic, social and cognitive knowledge (Roth and Spekman, 1984), is such that a disorder in pragmatics represents a deficit in linguistic/communicative, social and cognitive development. The language/communicative deficits already described in this chapter can be seen to underpin social difficulties. For example, difficulties with the interactive process in communication, in particular poor listening and communicative turn-taking, can cause students with a pragmatic disorder to appear egocentric and be unpopular with peers. Difficulties in interpreting contextual information can prevent children from distinguishing humour from serious comment. Therefore developing the aspects of language/communication affected by a pragmatic disorder will produce an impact on social development also.

Some of the ways in which the cognitive abilities of children with a pragmatic disorder can be disrupted have already been referred to, in particular their ability to plan and organize. Experience has also shown that the thinking styles of children with a pragmatic disorder appear to be rather narrow and inflexible, as encapsulated by the examples in Figure 3.5. It would seem reasonable to suggest that this style of thinking may be linked to the kinds of over-literal interpretation described earlier in this chapter. The second example in Figure 3.5 also shows a difficulty stemming from the misinterpretation of opinion as fact.

Children with a pragmatic disorder can do well on verbal IQ tests because these may not be sensitive to pragmatic aspects of language/communication. Pragmatic difficulties do occur in children with

Example 1. Context: *A teacher is demonstrating common materials, using different kinds of utensils. One of the utensils is a spoon. It is made of plastic, but is smooth and coloured in a way that gives an appearance of an animal's horns.*

Teacher: This spoon is made of plastic.
Child: (examining the spoon closely) It's horn.
Teacher: You mean it's like an animal's horns.
Child: Yes it's horn.
Teacher: Yes, it looks like an animal's horns, but this is plastic – we don't have spoons made of animal's horns (produces other examples of plastic and makes comparisons).
Child: (becoming frustrated) This is HORN!

Example 2. Context: *A teacher is describing the digestive system.*
Teacher: ...so what happens in the stomach and intestines is called digestion – it's the body taking what it needs from the food. The rest is waste, the body doesn't need it – and that's why we go to the toilet.
Child: It's poisonous.
Teacher: No, it's not poisonous, it's just waste – what the body doesn't need from the food.
Child: Jake (boy child likes) says it's poisonous.
Teacher: Well, Jake is wrong. It isn't poisonous, it's just what the body doesn't need from the food.
Child (becoming upset) It is poisonous!
Teacher: Well let's leave that now, we can talk about it again...

Figure 3.5 Examples to illustrate the 'narrow' thinking/learning styles in children with pragmatic disorders.

general learning difficulties and here IQ scores will be lower than average as a result of the more global learning difficulty. However, children who have primary pragmatic disorders (akin to those originally described as semantic–pragmatic disorder) can attain average scores on verbal and performance IQ subtests. In the next section, an urgent need will be identified for the inclusion of tests specifically focusing on pragmatics in screening assessment batteries; this includes those used by educational psychologists in determining statements of educational need.

The distinction between semantics and pragmatics

The examples cited in the previous section serve to illustrate a number of distinctions between the semantic and pragmatic areas. However, the difference between semantics and pragmatics appears to be seen as something of a 'grey area' in theoretical accounts of language. Whereas some theorists have considered pragmatics to be a distinct area, apart from semantics (Morris, 1938; Leech, 1983; Levinson, 1983), others have incorporated the notion of pragmatics within semantic theory (Kempson, 1977). Perhaps it is for this reason that an uncertainty about the distinction between semantics and pragmatics has pervaded practice.

However, in recent years there have been calls for pragmatics to be considered apart from semantics in describing children's language difficulties (McTear and Conti-Ramsden, 1992; Smith and Leinonen, 1992).

In the field of childhood language disorder, the notion of considering semantics and pragmatic difficulties together was perhaps most strongly influenced by Rapin and Allen's (1987) classification of language disorder: in particular, the inclusion of a term semantic–pragmatic syndrome. This term referred to children who exhibited deficits in abstract comprehension and in the formulation of discourse; they made atypical choices of words and inordinate use of scripts, and had a seeming lack of need for a conversational partner in their often verbose output (Rapin and Allen, 1998, p. 82).

Whilst this description brings the notion of pragmatic disorders to the fore, it raises problems with the term semantic–pragmatic syndrome (or semantic–pragmatic disorder; Bishop, 1989). For example, some of the features of the language of children described as semantic–pragmatic disorder by Rapin and Allen, in particular 'sophisticated vocabularies', indicate that in some sense the semantic area is a relative strength for these children. The author's experience is also that children referred as exhibiting semantic–pragmatic disorder, whilst having significant difficulty with the aspects of pragmatics described in the previous section, can do relatively well on tests of semantic comprehension and expressive vocabulary.

These points support McTear and Conti-Ramsden's (1992) view that the term semantic–pragmatic disorder obscures the nature of the difficulty it represents. The necessary co-occurrence of semantic and pragmatic difficulties suggested by the term may also obscure the process of identification. Pragmatic difficulties may remain undetected unless they are focused upon specifically in assessment. Difficulties in the areas of language selection/organization and pragmatic comprehension are particularly vulnerable to missed detection because they present relatively late in communication development, usually after the child has entered school. The importance of special needs coordinators remaining attuned to the nature of pragmatic deficits would appear paramount here.

The development of assessments to tap pragmatic difficulties appears to have fallen behind other language areas. In 1992, reviews by Smith and Leinonen and McTear and Conti-Ramsden identified a number of observation checklists to assess the interactive process of communication. However, it is only in recent years that the assessment of pragmatic processing in comprehension and language selection/organization has begun to be specifically addressed (for example, Wiig, 1988; Rinaldi, 1996, 1999). There is scope for much further development here, in particular in the area of standardized procedures. It is vitally important that pragmatic assessments are included in screening measures and that users are clear of the distinction between pragmatics and semantics. For example, misinterpretation may arise in the assessment of children's figurative language. It has already been noted that the exploration of the comprehension of idiomatic expression and other forms of figurative language cannot tap pragmatic processing unless items are presented in context. Assessments of pragmatic comprehension also need to include a way of indicating whether children can detect their own miscomprehension, since this provides a useful pragmatic strategy that can be taught if necessary.

Finally, the current use of terminology is very misleading, both to parents and professionals, as encapsulated by this extract, from a lecture on pragmatic disorder given by the author in 1998:

> Children with particular difficulties in pragmatics are sometimes called semantic–pragmatic disorder, but it is actually the pragmatic area which presents the greatest difficulty within the language profile. There are children who do have significant difficulties with both the semantic and the pragmatic areas (they may also have difficulty, or a history of difficulty, with phonology and grammar), but the term semantic–pragmatic disorder isn't applied to this type of difficulty – this type of difficulty is referred to as language disorder.

Based on the points raised in this section, the proposal of this chapter is that children previously described as exhibiting semantic–pragmatic disorder could more accurately be described under the category of a pragmatic disorder.

Consideration will now be given of how to consider those with a pragmatic disorder in relation to other special needs groups. The following section, in particular, explores the similarities and differences between a pragmatic disorder, specific developmental language disorder (SDLD) and autism.

Pragmatic disorder, SDLD and autism

Introduction

The main objective in exploring the similarities and differences between pragmatic disorder, SDLD and autism is to consider whether or when pragmatic disorders are most usefully viewed a) as a form of language disorder or b) as a form of autism. The question whether pragmatic disorders can be most usefully located within an autism context can be seen as arising because of the position of pragmatics at the interface between linguistic, cognitive and social knowledge (Roth and Spekman, 1984). Pragmatics represents an aspect of language that is essentially to do with communication and, therefore, essentially social. Autism has been identified as primarily a social deficit (Wing, 1988): communication difficulties emanate from this core deficit. Developmental language disorder is primarily a linguistic deficit which can impact upon social development (Griffiths, 1969; Haynes and Naidoo, 1991). A central question of the language disorder/ autism debate therefore concerns the primacy of pragmatic disorder: linguistic or social? A further area of exploration could be in comparing the cognitive deficits in the autism and language disorder contexts. These questions will be returned to later in this chapter.

At this point the reader may well ask: *What does it matter?* The author has some sympathy with this viewpoint: in a sense, the key issues are to acknowledge the existence of a pragmatic disorder, to have the tools to identify the difficulty and the resources to do something about it, regardless of whether it occurs as a form of SDLD or a form of autism. However, there may be considerable implications arising from the ways in which parents, practitioners and managers in education come to view this kind of difficulty. Boucher (1998) for example, proposes implications for prognosis, educational placement and intervention:

> The long-term prognosis for children with specific language impairment is generally better than for children with autism … In autism, normal reciprocal relationships cannot be made and independent living is possible only for a small minority. If SPD (semantic–pragmatic disorder[4]) is a specific language disorder characterized by impaired learning and use of linguistic forms and meanings, therapy should be directed at remedial language teaching and conversational uses of language. If SPD is allied to autism then therapy and management will have a broader set of aims and methods. If SPD is a form of specific language impairment then placement in a language unit or special school for language impaired children may be appropriate. If SPD is a form of autism then placement in an autistic class or special school for children with autism may be appropriate (p. 72).

The author has further experienced the view that, when pragmatic disorders are associated with autism or Asperger's syndrome, an appropriate placement is a special school for children with emotional/behavioural difficulties, because of the primacy of the personal social impairment in these conditions.

---

[4] Refers to the condition described in this chapter as pragmatic disorder

With these implications in mind, pragmatic disorders will first be considered in the context of developmental language disorder. The current and historical perspectives on autism and Asperger's syndrome will then be summarized as a background to considering pragmatic disorders in the context of autism.

Pragmatic disorders in the context of developmental language disorder

Boucher (1998) states that if 'semantic–pragmatic disorder'[5] is to be established as a sub-type of SDLD, then it must be shown to resemble other sub-types of SDLD in involving language system acquisition difficulties, but reliable differences must also be shown to exist between the language acquisition difficulties in pragmatic disorders and other sub-types of SDLD.

There is some research evidence to indicate similarities between a pragmatic disorder and SDLD, for example in comprehension of inferential and ambiguous meaning (Bishop and Adams, 1992; Rinaldi, 2000). Rinaldi proposes that the children in her sample may have had difficulty in resolving ambiguity because of deficiencies in processing at both the language and metacognitive levels. Further study may explore similarities and differences in these kinds of processing between pragmatic disorders and other sub-types of SDLD.

Comparing the pragmatic expressive abilities of children with SDLD and pragmatic disorder, Bishop and Adams (1989) found no difference in conversational exchange structure and repairs, but they did find that children with pragmatic disorders made more initiations than SDLD children. There may be further qualitative differences here if, for example, differences in turn-taking are exacerbated by poor word retention in SDLD. In other words, if the child is unable to express his or her ideas at the time of processing them (which may coincide with a time when someone else is speaking) they may not be able to express them at all. In pragmatic disorder, turn-taking difficulties may be more to do with metacommunicative awareness.

Studies into SDLD children's expressive pragmatic abilities, as compared with those of non-impaired children, have been inconclusive. For example, Brinton et al. (1986) found SDLD children used the same range of speech acts (requesting, commenting, responding and clarifying) as non-impaired language age peers. Rowan et al. (1983) found that SDLD children construct equally informative messages by 'foregrounding' new information and 'backgrounding' old information. Brinton and Fujiki

---

[5] Refers to the condition described in this chapter as pragmatic disorder.

(1982), however, found that SDLD children produced fewer requests for clarification than non-impaired children and Craig and Evans (1989) found that SDLD children made more conversational interruptions.

In Chapter 1 it was noted that pragmatic difficulties in SDLD are more prominent in the secondary school years, on account of the relatively late onset of pragmatic skills in normal development and the changing demands on children as they grow older. Since pragmatic disorders do not show themselves fully until the secondary school years, it would appear important to study this age group if we are to most accurately explore similarities and differences between pragmatic disorders and sub-types of SDLD.

There is also some anecdotal evidence, from the author's assessment of junior and secondary school-aged children, that some SDLD children can demonstrate the 'narrow thinking styles' evident in children with pragmatic disorders. This kind of thinking style may reflect the general effects of a specific learning difficulty; that is, because learning is effortful, there is a tendency for children to over-generalize points of learning. Over-literal interpretation (of visual and auditory information) and the ability to distinguish fact from opinion can also be a feature of SDLD children's cognitive style. The inability to plan hierarchically has been identified as an area of cognitive dysfunction in SDLD children (Cromer, 1983). It may be proposed that difficulties with language coherence, frequently impaired in pragmatic disorder in ways outlined earlier in this chapter, could be linked to a cognitive dysfunction of this kind.

The differences between language acquisition in pragmatic disorder and SDLD may concern the pattern or degree of disruption. Vance (1993), for example, suggests that:

> some of the features found in the language of children within the sub-group of semantic pragmatic disorder[6] may be common to all children with specific language impairment, but are more noticeable and more noted in this sub-group, because all other aspects of language are relatively intact (p. 5).

The proposal here is that in pragmatic disorder there are greater difficulties per se with pragmatics and also a greater discrepancy of difficulty compared with the remaining language profile. That is, difficulty with elements of language acquisition concerning pragmatic processing may be shared in pragmatic disorder and (other) types of SDLD, to various degrees, but the difficulties with elements of language acquisition affecting areas outside the pragmatic domain are not shared. There may also be differences in the pattern of difficulty: whereas in pragmatic

---

[6] Refers to the condition described in this chapter as pragmatic disorder.

disorder all aspects of pragmatic ability may be affected, in SDLD only certain aspects may be impaired. Tentative evidence for this proposal comes from the varying findings of research, cited above, into SDLD children's abilities across the range of pragmatic areas studied.

Further investigation is needed to confirm similarities and differences in the deficits of the language (and cognitive) systems and processes underpinning pragmatic disorder and SDLD. It will be important to explore areas of comprehension, expression and communicative interaction to account for differences in pattern of difficulty.

A first step in this investigation may be to develop an assessment battery to provide a more accurate comparison across the language profile. A paucity of pragmatic assessments and in particular standardized pragmatic assessments has already been identified. There is a serious gap in our knowledge with regard to the normal developmental process across pragmatic areas: normative research is particularly lacking in the area of language selection and organization. Currently it is difficult to make comprehensive language-age related comparisons across linguistic profiles (taking in aspects of phonology, grammar, semantics and pragmatics) and across pragmatic profiles (taking in aspects of comprehension, language selection/organization and communicative interaction).

In the introduction to this section, key considerations in determining where pragmatic disorders 'best fit' in the language disorder or autism contexts concerned intervention, educational placement and prognosis. The author is aware from her experience that a language-based, metacognitive approach (described in Chapter 4) can have significant effects for children with pragmatic disorder and can ultimately shift the prognosis for these children. The author's experience is also that teaching groups comprising children with pragmatic disorders and children with specific language disorders (where pragmatic difficulties form part of the disorder, and are not so severe) are more effective than teaching groups comprising children who all have pragmatic disorders. This finding may be a reflection of the balance between similarities and differences in the two disorders; that is, there is enough similarity to enable effective teaching for children with both types of disorder, but differences which enable them to learn from each other's strengths. Clearly, formal research needs to be conducted to support these observations. Botting (1998) says that children with pragmatic disorders move much more slowly in and out of language provision than other children with language disorders. However, this picture may shift as practitioners develop a better understanding and improved teaching methods to focus on the pragmatic area. In the past, this has been difficult because pragmatics has arrived late in our awareness of children's language difficulties. In 1987, for example, study in the field of pragmatic disorder was declared to be in a state of infancy (Fey and Leonard, 1983). It was not until 1992 that the first comprehensive texts on childhood pragmatic disorders were published in the UK (McTear and Conti-Ramsden, 1992 ; Smith and Leinonen, 1992). Pragmatics also represents a relatively abstract aspect of language that can appear 'intangible' to teaching activity. However, ways in which the 'intangibility' can be converted into the concrete domain are increasingly coming to the fore (for example, Bell, 1991; Rinaldi, 1992, 1995, 1996a, 1999; Kelly, 1996).

Knowledge in the field of pragmatics is continually developing. The view expressed in this book is that past difficulties in locating pragmatic disorder in relation to language disorder/autism have arisen because insufficient attention and appreciation has been given to pragmatics and the language disorder context. This is evident in some of the statements made about developmental language disorders by researchers who believe that pragmatic disorder is a sub-type of autism (or, most recently, pervasive developmental disorder). For example, *we do not know whether it is possible for a child to be communicatively impaired yet unimpaired socially and symbolically. We would argue that it is – children with developmental language disorder are a good example of this* (Brook and Bowler, 1998, p. 94). However, the social difficulties of children with developmental language disorders are well documented (Griffiths, 1969; Haynes and Naidoo, 1991; Roux, 1997). Difficulties in symbolic understanding as a feature of developmental language disorder have also been documented (Cooper et al., 1978; Roth and Clark, 1987; Udwin and Yule, 1983).

It can be argued that the DSM-IV classification of developmental language disorder (American Psychiatric Association, 1994) has fallen considerably behind theoretical accounts of language (as summarized by the definitions in Figure 3.1) by not including pragmatic disorder in this classification. Interestingly, the American Speech and Language Association does include pragmatic difficulties in its definition of language disorder.

It was proposed at the beginning of this chapter that attempts to view pragmatic disorder in the context of autism may have gathered momentum because pragmatics represents a position at the interface of linguistic, social and cognitive knowledge (Roth and Spekman, 1994). However, this interface position does not divorce pragmatics from the linguistic picture and does not identify a primacy to the social deficit. Pragmatic skills rely heavily upon linguistic (syntactic and semantic) context, as demonstrated earlier in this chapter. Where pragmatics concerns non-linguistic context, the interest is upon the interaction between non-linguistic and linguistic factors.

There may be some cases of pragmatic disorder that could be more helpfully viewed within the context of autism (or, according to the DSM-IV revised, pervasive developmental disorder) and possible indicators will be included in subsequent sections. However, it is argued here that to view pragmatic disorder exclusively within the context of autism, as proposed by authors such as Brook and Bowler (1992, 1998) and Happe (1994), is to serve a major injustice to the children with pragmatic disorders and their parents, in terms of the appropriate intervention approaches that may be offered to them and, ultimately, in terms of their prognosis. The author's practice suggests that the prognosis of children with pragmatic disorders, given the appropriate intervention, is far better than that outlined by Boucher for autism: *In autism, normal reciprocal relationships cannot be made and independent living is possible for only a very small minority*.

It seems valid to conclude that the most effective focus of intervention for children with pragmatic disorder is linguistic–cognitive. It is the development of underlying language/communicative and cognitive processing that enables children with pragmatic disorders to be more effective socially. This focus may actually also apply to pragmatic disorders in the context of autism (or pervasive developmental disorders), but as Boucher (1998) identifies, there may be a broader focus to intervention here.

Perspectives on autism and Asperger's syndrome

Autism

Kanner's (1943) first account of autism, based on the observations of 11 children, included the following characteristic features:

* **Inability to relate** to people

* **Failure to develop speech or largely non-communicative** use of language ... obsessive questioning and ritualistic use of language

* Behaviour governed by an **obsessive desire for sameness**

* Good cognitive potential with **excellent rote memory**

Kanner's account presents autism as a syndrome: a unified condition with a single cause and a symptom pattern that tends towards being the same in all cases (Boucher, 1998). Since this first account, the description of autism has undergone a number of developments that emphasize the variability of the condition (Frith, 1989; American Psychiatric Association, 1994). Autism has been described as a continuum of disorders, emphasizing degrees of pattern or severity (Wing, 1988) and, with greater popularity in more recent times, as a spectrum of related disorder 'sub-types' (revised DSM-IV). There is less emphasis on the inability to relate to people (Frith, 1989); however, social impairment has been identified as the core impairment of autism (Wing, 1988).

This change of perspective represents a shift away from considering autism in terms of symptoms, as outlined by Kanner, towards considering autism in terms of difficulties underpinning three areas or the 'triad of impairment' (Wing, 1988; Frith, 1989):

- The capacity to form and maintain sophisticated social relationships
- Intentional communication
- Imaginative activity

Frith proposed the underlying difficulties of this triad of impairments to be in the area of cognitive functioning, for example, in the ability to make 'second order representations': that is, the ability to know that something can function as something else. Frith also proposes that autistic individuals have impaired ability to mentalize (after Premack's Theory of Mind); that is, to attribute mental states with content to others.

The changes in perspectives on autism have been reflected in the DSM-IV (American Psychiatric Association, 1994), an internationally recognized set of diagnostic criteria for mental and behaviour disorders. In the most recent revision, however, the general term 'autism' has been replaced by 'pervasive developmental disorder'. The term 'autistic disorder' is used only to refer to the original concept of autism as outlined by Kanner, as one sub-type of a 'pervasive developmental disorder'. The other sub-types specified are 'Asperger disorder' (previously termed Asperger's syndrome) Retts disorder, 'childhood disintegrative disorder' and 'pervasive developmental disorder not otherwise specified'.

In a sense, the move back to using the term 'autism' as originally conceptualized is helpful from both practical and research perspectives. The use of the term had been stretched so far that it had become impossible to know whether a reference to autism in a report or research paper, represented a group of children with an inability to relate to people and an uncommunicative use of language, as described by Kanner, or a group of children with social impairments as described by Wing and Frith. Clearly the type and level of resourcing needed for these groups of children is very different.

However, the term 'pervasive developmental disorder' has not yet been widely adopted in the UK; perhaps out of fear of muddying the waters further: there is already inconsistency in how the terms 'autism', 'Asperger's syndrome', 'semantic–pragmatic disorder' are used in the UK (Bishop, 1989). The notion of 'pervasive developmental disorder not otherwise specified' may appear rather vague and there may be a concern from practitioners that such a term could become a 'diagnostic dumping ground'.

Regardless of the terms used, a question that may be asked is *has sufficient scrutiny been given to the validity of extending the original notion of autism?* This returns to what in the author's view is the central issue underlying the autism/language disorder debate: the primacy of disorder amongst the interwoven areas of language, social and cognitive knowledge. In autism, the social deficit is primary (Wing and Gould, 1979; Wing, 1988); in SDLD the language disorder is the primary deficit. In both disorders there are deficits to cognitive processing: there may be differences and overlaps here. Kanner's description of autism included excellent rote memory, which is not a feature of SDLD. However, other cognitive deficits identified in the extended view of autism, such as difficulty with second order representation, may also be evident in children with language disorder. For example, limited imaginative play has been identified as a feature of developmental language delay/disorder emanating from a delay in the development of symbolic understanding (Cooper et al., 1978; McCune-Nicholich, 1981; Tallal, 1988). Udwin and Yule (1983) and Roth and Clark (1987) uncovered significant differences in the complexity of symbolic play between children with receptive language disorders and non-impaired groups.

The extended view of autism may be useful to identify a group of children who have primary social deficits but who display some or all of the pragmatic difficulties evident in pragmatic disorder. For example, Rapin and Allen (1998) point to unusual perseveration and preoccupations in interests (in addition to disordered communication) to distinguish autism from pragmatic disorders in the language disorder context. This aspect of behaviour can be viewed as relating to Kanner's description 'obsessive desire for sameness'. A note of caution here is that children with developmental language disorders can also have a poor awareness or a narrow range of interests. For example, it may be that a tendency to favour a particular interest arises from a feeling of insecurity bound up with the general psychological effects of a language/communication difficulty. However, an 'obsession' with particular interests is not usually a feature of developmental language disorder.

In some cases, it may be virtually impossible to disentangle deficits in social, language and cognitive development to determine primacy of disorder. However, from an intervention viewpoint, matters, fortunately, may be less complex. Here, experience has shown that a focus on pragmatic language – in the receptive and expressive domains – can provide a very useful mechanism for developing social knowledge in children with autism (in the extended view) (Aarons and Gittens, 1998) and language disorder (Rinaldi, 1992, 1996).

The study of the social effects of pragmatic language intervention in children with autism-related disorders (or sub-types of pervasive developmental disorder) is clearly an area where research is badly needed in order to more rigorously advocate a language-based approach for these children.

Asperger's syndrome

Asperger's original account of the disorder appears similar to autism: deficient social behaviour; obsessional interests; pedantic, stereotyped speech and clumsiness. There has been some argument over whether the overlap between Asperger's syndrome and autism merits consideration of Asperger's syndrome as a distinct category. However, it has been argued that the prognosis for children with Asperger's syndrome is more favourable than autism (Wing, 1981; Howlin, 1987), and Asperger's syndrome has been identified as a synonym for autism of a less severe kind (Schopler, 1985).

Bishop (1989) notes that it is not only the severity of disorder but also the pattern of symptoms that differ between autism and Asperger's syndrome. A feature of Asperger's syndrome is that verbal IQ is well above performance IQ (Wing, 1981). The advanced verbal skills of children with Asperger's syndrome is also emphasized by Tantum's description (1988): autistic people who are sociable, highly clumsy, verbally skilled and with highly developed special interests.

Despite their verbal strengths, children with Asperger's syndrome do have communication deficits. Gillberg and Gillberg (1989) noted 'unusual speech and language' to include superficially perfect expressive language, formal pedantic language, and impairments of comprehension including misinterpretation of implied meanings.

The author's experience is that the *superficially perfect expressive language* comes about because of advanced linguistic skills at word and sentence level (in both comprehension and expression). This can give a false first impression of communicative competence. On continued conversation, difficulties with relevance and coherence become evident. That is, children with Asperger's syndrome are able to construct meaningful utterances, with understanding (in contrast to echolalia, where a phrase or sentence is repeated without meaning), but are unaware of appropriate selection and organization of language in a communicative context, in particular, with reference to listener need. These kinds of difficulties were described earlier in this chapter as a feature of pragmatic disorder that occurs as a function of poor language-choice making. Attwood's (1998) description of children with Asperger's syndrome alludes to these types of difficulty: 'the child may talk too much or too little ... garrulous speech, a never ending "babbling brook" ... In contrast, some children may have periods when they are genuinely "lost for words".'

The advanced expressive and receptive language skills at word and sentence level can also mask serious comprehension deficits at the pragmatic level. Children with Asperger's syndrome can make over-literal interpretations that affect comprehension of sarcasm, jest and figurative language. The difficulty is not in learning multiple meanings per se, but in comprehending which meaning is intended. The author has some evidence that children with Asperger's syndrome may be able to use their advanced skills at word and sentence level to work out intended meanings in figurative language, without understanding the underlying pragmatic function. As stated earlier in this chapter, levels of pragmatic processing needed to resolve ambiguous meaning include plausibility judgement, detection of miscomprehension and awareness of the need to seek alternative referents. The author has recorded instances where children with Asperger's syndrome have been able to determine multiple or idiomatic meanings presented in context. However, further exploration (the children were asked why they hadn't selected the literal interpretation as speaker intention) revealed that the children had used syntactic congruity to determine speaker intention as opposed to making plausibility judgements as non-impaired children do (Rinaldi, 2000). For example, when asked why a road covered in strawberry jam had not been selected as the speaker's meaning in the utterance 'I'm sorry I'm late the road was jammed solid this morning', a student with Asperger's syndrome (CA 12;6) reported: 'the verb jam means a traffic jam, strawberry jam is a noun so this one (pointing to picture of road covered in strawberry jam) didn't work'. Further exploration is required to examine whether such instances are evident in other children with Asperger's syndrome and whether this may provide a feature of Asperger's syndrome as distinct from other kinds of pragmatic disorder.

The difficulties children with Asperger's syndrome have in making over-literal interpretation transcends the domain of language: they can also misread situations. The inflexibility/narrowness of thinking style referred to in children with pragmatic disorders appears particularly marked. As Attwood (1998) relates: 'their thinking tends to be rigid and not to adapt to change or failure. They may have only one approach to a problem and need tuition in thinking of alternatives'. Attwood identifies a consequence of this difficulty as an inability to learn from mistakes: this feature can clearly affect learning progress and needs to be addressed specifically in teaching approaches.

The difficulties children with Asperger's syndrome have in adapting to change or failure can also cause them considerable frustration and anxiety and this can lead to problems with social behaviour. Figure 3.6 outlines two examples of this. In each instance, developing an understanding of concepts underpinning the difficulty in reading the situation (in the first

---

Example 1

I watched Pan in the playground. Another boy ran passed him – his jacket was blown open by the wind and caught Pan's face. I saw Pan run after the boy and thump him in the back. Pan's interpretation was that the boy had deliberately hurt him, when in fact it had clearly been an accident.

Later that term Pan was found stamping on another boy's bag, in floods of tears. He was in a terrible state, virtually inconsolable. It transpired the bag had fallen from a shelf – the contents had scattered – a lucky mascot treasured by the bag's owner was broken. A number of boys, including Pan, were in the classroom at the time. Pan was adamant that he wasn't responsible for the bag and set about proving it! (He showed the teacher a drawing he had been working on at the time of the incident.) Nevertheless, because no one owned up to the incident they were all kept in for a short detention. This meant that Pan missed most of his favourite TV programme.

Pan's inability to manage this incident arose because of his inability to manage what he perceived to be extremely unjust. None of the others were happy about the detention but they accepted the teacher's decision. The general view was that it was only a short detention so it wasn't worth making a fuss about.

Example 2

Jag was referred at the age of 17. He had had a number of 'bad experiences' at school resulting in one exclusion. His parents had recently withdrawn him from a second school. Jag told me that he had done some 'silly things' for his friends. It transpired that some other students had persuaded him to break school rules and to put himself in considerable danger. Jag considered these students to be his friends, agreeing to do as they asked as a strategy for friendship.

Figure 3.6 Examples of difficulty in interpretation in two children with Asperger's syndrome.[7]

---

[7] For reasons of confidentiality, the names of the children have been changed.

example the concept of accident/on purpose and the concept of fairness; in the second the concept of bullying in contrast to 'true friendship') helped the students. Alternative strategies to aggressive/fearful responses were then introduced.

Identifying the communication difficulties of children with Asperger's syndrome can be problematic. Their difficulties may not be evident in the preschool period. Bishop (1989) reports normal language development in the early years; Gillberg and Gillberg (1989) note that any delay in language development appears to have been caught up by the time the child enters school.

Managing children with Asperger's syndrome requires considerable skill and a full understanding of their problems. If not understood, their difficulties can be perceived as a behaviour problem: the difficulties in thinking and learning can be so at odds with their 'superficially perfect language' that practitioners can be left feeling that their learning and social behaviour is wilful or attention-seeking. The examples in Figure 3.6. indicate how deficits in pragmatic comprehension and cognitive style can easily manifest as a 'behaviour problem'.

Children with Asperger's syndrome often start their education in a mainstream school (in the private or public sector) but their difficulties usually become evident in the junior school years. Mainstream staff not aware of the nature of deficit can feel ill-equipped to deal with these very specific difficulties, and there is a strong training need here. The mainstream context can provide a good learning and social experience for children with Asperger's syndrome if (and it's a pretty hefty 'if') staff have the necessary understanding and skills to manage the children's learning and social development. Indeed, often the children have a strong desire to attend their local school with peers of equal intellect. However, the consequences of children attending mainstream schools where staff are not adequately trained can be very serious. The educational approach needs to include specific teaching on thinking and learning strategies and on the management of social situations.

Pragmatic disorder and Asperger's syndrome

Children with Asperger's syndrome tend to have superior linguistic skills at word and sentence level (hence their superficially perfect speech) compared to children with pragmatic disorder, but they share difficulties in interpreting implied meaning and relevance/coherence. This is not to say that children with pragmatic disorder have particular difficulties at word or sentence level, but children with Asperger's syndrome can have verbal IQs well above average. Children with Asperger's syndrome may do better than children with pragmatic disorders on tests of non-literal interpretation because, as outlined in the preceding section, they may use their superior linguistic skills to compensate for deficits in pragmatic processing, sometimes successfully.

The author's experience is that thinking styles of children with Asperger's syndrome and pragmatic disorder bear similarity, but the inflexibility is more marked in Asperger's syndrome. The author's view is that it is this part of the profile of difficulty that can restrict progress, and the prognosis of Asperger syndrome may therefore be poorer than pragmatic disorder. However, as our knowledge and competence in developing thinking styles improves, the outlook for children with Asperger's syndrome (and pragmatic disorder) should be on an upward turn.

Developmental impairments: continua vs. sub-types

In Chapter 1 the difficulties in describing special needs, in particular developmental language disorder, in terms of sub-types were discussed. It was suggested that the use of sub-types may be limiting, and not reflect the various permutations seen under the umbrella of developmental language disorder.

Variations and overlaps *across* conditions, for example, 'developmental language disorder', 'autism', and 'general learning difficulties', also seems apparent. For example, terms heard in day-to-day practice include 'MLD plus'; 'bit autistic' 'autisticky', 'more than a language disorder', and 'a touch language disordered', to name but a few.

Boucher (1998) discusses the usefulness of considering developmental impairments as continua as opposed to sub-types. She notes that the word 'continuum' connotes variety introduced by degrees of severity and has a strong practical value in its power to explain the heterogeneity of developmental disorders. Boucher refers to autism (with reference to Wing, 1988) and developmental language disorder, in particular. However, the notion of continua may be useful across a range of special needs. Viewing developmental disorders as a series of overlapping continua may facilitate a clearer understanding of both pattern and degree of difficulty. For example, continua of learning difficulty, cognitive styles, language/communication difficulty and social behaviour could be helpful in accounting for the various overlaps and permutations seen when working with children who have 'moderate learning difficulties', 'Asperger's syndrome', 'specific developmental language disorder', etc.

Conclusion

Pragmatics has been identified as an area of linguistic study, either separate from semantics or subsumed within semantic theory. There is evidence from theoretical, clinical and educational perspectives of a need to consider pragmatics apart from semantics. Pragmatic difficulties occur commonly in children with SDLD and are particularly evident in the secondary school years, contributing to difficulties in social development in this group. Children with pragmatic disorder, who have more marked and specific pragmatic difficulties (in relation to the remaining language profile), can learn well alongside children with broader-ranging language difficulties. These factors indicate a justification and educational value in considering pragmatic disorder in a context of language disorder.

Pragmatic disorder can also occur alongside other factors that indicate a more primary social deficit, as in the case of the extended view of autism and Asperger's syndrome. Factors highlighted have included 'preoccupations' and perseveration with particular interests, and a lack of social imagination/imaginative play. It was noted that SDLD children can also have a restricted range/knowledge of interests and lack imagination in play, but there may be qualitative differences here.

In Asperger's syndrome it is perhaps the cognitive dysfunction, in particular relating to inflexible thinking styles, that is the strongest feature, alongside advanced verbal skills at word and sentence level. Of the sub-types of autism (or pervasive developmental disorders) Asperger's syndrome (or Asperger disorder) possibly bears the strongest resemblance to pragmatic disorder; however the cognitive deficit is more marked and this, together with the superior verbal skills shifts the emphasis away from the linguistic deficit. Nevertheless, communicative difficulties, whilst perhaps not being immediately evident, are considerable, and form an important part of the profile of disorder in identification and intervention.

This chapter has focused upon pragmatic disorder in the contexts of SDLD and autism; however, pragmatic difficulties are not exclusive to these groups. For example, children with specific difficulties in written language can have problems with language selection and organization that become evident in creative writing. Visually impaired children may be particularly vulnerable to faulty interaction skills because they do not pick up on visual non-verbal cues. Comparison of pragmatic ability across special needs groups and the underlying deficits contributing to the observed difficulties is an area worthy of much further research. The position of pragmatics at the interface of social, cognitive and linguistic knowledge is such that of all the aspects of language difficulty it is likely to have the most far-reaching of consequences when it goes wrong, and the most far-reaching of consequences when it is put right.

References

Aarons M, Gittens T. Autism: A Social Skills Approach. Oxford: Winslow Press, 1998.

Ackerman B. On comprehending idioms: Do children get the picture? Journal of Experimental Psychology 1982; 33: 439–54.

American Psychiatric Association. Diagnostic and Statistical Manual of Mental Disorders (3rd revised edition) (DSM-IV). Washington, DC: American Psychiatric Association, 1994.

Attwood AJ. Asperger's Syndrome. London: Jessica Kingsley, 1998.

Bell, N. Visualizing and Verbalizing. California: Academy of Reading Publications, 1991.

Bishop DVM. Autism, Asperger's syndrome and semantic–pragmatic disorder: where are the boundaries? British Journal of Disorders of Communication 1989; 24: 107–21.

Bishop DVM, Adams C. Conversational characteristics of children with semantic–pragmatic disorder II. What features lead to a judgement of inappropriacy? British Journal of Disorders of Communication 1989; 24: 241–63.

Bishop DVM, Adams C. Comprehension problems in children with specific language impairment: literal and inferential meaning. Journal of Speech and Hearing Research 1992; 35: 119–29.

Bloom L, Lahey M. Language Development and Language Disorders. London: John Wiley and Sons, 1978.

Botting N. Semantic–pragmatic disorder as a distinct diagnostic entity: making sense of the boundaries. International Journal of Language and Communication Disorders 1998; 33 (1): 87–91.

Boucher J. SPD as a distinct diagnostic entity: logical considerations and directions for future research. International Journal of Language and Communication Disorders 1998; 33: 1.

Brinton B, Fujiki M. A comparison of request–response sequences in the discourse of normal and language-disordered children. Journal of Speech and Hearing Disorders 1982; 47: 57–62.

Brinton B, Fujiki M, Winkler E, Loeb D. Responses to requests for clarification in linguistically normal and language-impaired children. Journal of Speech and Hearing Disorders 1986; 51: 370–8.

Brook SL, Bowler DM. Autism by another name? Semantic and pragmatic impairments in children. Journal of Autism and Developmental Disorders 1992; 22: 61–81.

Brook SL, Bowler DM. SPD and autism spectrum disorder. International Journal of Language and Communication Disorders 1998; 33: 1.

Cacciari C, Levorato M. How children understand idioms in discourse. Journal of Child Language 1989; 16: 387–405.

Cooper J, Moodley M, Reynell J. Helping Language Development. London: Edward Arnold, 1978.

Craig H, Evans J. Turn exchange characteristics of SLI children's simultaneous speech. Journal of Speech and Language Disorders 1989; 54: 334–47.

Cromer R. Hierarchical planning disability in the drawings and constructions of a group of severely dysphasic children. Brain and Cognition 1983; 2: 144–64.

Crystal D. Concept of language development: A realistic perspective. In Rule R, Rutter M (eds) Language Development and Language Disorders. London: MacKeith Press, 1987.

Fey ME, Leonard LB. Pragmatic skills of children with specific language impairment. In Gallagher TM, Prutting CA (eds) Pragmatic Assessment and Intervention Issues in Language. San Diego, CA: College Hill Press, 1983.

Frith U. A new look at language and communication in autism. British Journal of Disorders of Communication 1989; 24: 123–50.

Gillberg C, Gillberg C. Asperger's syndrome – some epidemiological considerations: research note. Journal of Child Psychology and Psychiatry 1989; 30: 631–8.

Grice H. Logic and conversation. In Cole P, Morgan J (eds) Syntax and Semantics 3: Speech Acts. New York: Academic Press, 1975.

Griffiths C. A follow up study of children with articulation and language disorders. British Journal of Disorders of Communication 1969; 4: 46–56.

Happe F. Autism: An Introduction to Psychological Theory. London: UCL Press, 1994.

Haynes C, Naidoo S. Children with specific speech and language impairment. Clinics in Developmental Medicine No 119. London: MacKeith Press, 1991.

Howlin P. Asperger's syndrome – does it exist and what can be done about it? In Proceedings of the First International Symposium on Specific Speech and Language Disorders in Children. London: AFASIC, 1987.

Kanner L. Autistic disturbances of affective contact. Nervous Child 2217–250, 1943. Reprinted in Kanner L. Childhood Psychosis: Initial Studies and New Insights. New York: Wiley, 1973.

Kelly A. Talkabout: A Social Communication Skills Package. Oxford: Winslow Press Ltd, 1996.

Kempson RM. Semantic Theory. Cambridge: Cambridge University Press, 1977.

Kirchner D, Skarakis-Doyle E. Developmental language disorders: a theoretical perspective. In Gallagher T, Prutting C (eds) Pragmatic Assessment and Intervention Issues in Language. San Diego, CA: College Hill Press, 1983.

Leech G. Pragmatics. London: Longman Press, 1983.

Levinson S. Pragmatics. Cambridge: Cambridge University Press, 1983.

McCune-Nicholich L. Towards symbolic functioning. Structure of early pretend games and potential parallels with language. Child Development 1981; 52: 785–97.

McTear M, Conti-Ramsden G. Pragmatic Disability in Children. London: Whurr Publishers Ltd, 1992.

Morris C. Foundations of the theory of signs. In International Encyclopaedia of Unified Science, No. 2. Chicago: University of Chicago Press, 1938.

Rapin I, Allen DA. Developmental language disorders: nosologic considerations. In Kirk U (ed) Neuropsychology of Language, Reading and Spelling. New York: Academic Press, 1987.

Rapin I, Allen DA. The semantic–pragmatic deficit disorder: classification issues. International Journal of Language and Communication Disorders 1998; 33 (1): 82–7.

Rinaldi WF. The Social Use of Language Programme. Windsor: NFER Nelson, 1992.

Rinaldi WF. The Social Use of Language Programme – Primary and Infant School. Guildford: Child Communication and Learning, 1995.

Rinaldi WF. Social Use of Language Programme Storypack for College and Adult Students. Guildford: Child Communication and Learning, 1996.

Rinaldi WF. Understanding Ambiguity: An Assessment of Pragmatic Meaning Comprehension. Windsor: NFER-Nelson, 1996a.

Rinaldi WF. The inner life of youngsters with specific developmental language disorder. In Varma V (ed) The Inner Life of Children with Special Needs. London: Whurr Publishers Ltd, 1996b.

Rinaldi, WF. Language Choices. Guildford: Child Communication and Learning, 1999.

Rinaldi WF. Pragmatic comprehension in secondary school aged students with specific developmental language disorder. International Journal of Language and Communication Disorders 2000; 52: 1–29.

Roth F, Clark D. Symbolic play and social participation abilities of language impaired and normally developing children. Journal of Speech and Hearing Research 1987; 52: 17–29.

Roth F, Spekman N. Assessing the pragmatic abilities of children Part 1. Organizational framework and assessment parameters. Journal of Speech and Hearing Disorders 1984; 49: 2–11.

Roux J. Working with 11–16 year old pupils with language and communication difficulties in the mainstream school. Child Language, Teaching and Therapy 1997; 13 (3): 228–43.

Rowan L, Leonard L, Chapman K, Weiss A. Performative and presuppositional skills in language disordered and normal children. Journal of Speech and Hearing Research 1983; 26: 97–106.

Rustin L, Kuhr A. Social Skills and the Speech Impaired. London: Whurr Publishers Ltd, 1989.

Schopler E. Editorial: Convergence of learning disability, higher level autism and Asperger's syndrome. Journal of Autism and Developmental Disorders 1985; 15: 359.

Smith RB, Leinonen E. Clinical Pragmatics: Unravelling the Complexities of Communicative Failure. London: Chapman & Hall, 1992.

Tallal P. Developmental language disorders. In Kavanagh J, Truss T Jr (eds) Learning Disabilities: Proceedings of the National Conference. Parkton, MD: New York Press, 1988.

Tantum D. Asperger's syndrome. Journal of Child Psychology and Psychiatry 1988; 29: 245–55.

Udwin O, Yule W. Imaginative play in language disordered children. British Journal of Disorders of Communication 1983; 18 (3): 197–205.

Vance M. An investigation of non-iteral comprehension and recognition of intonation patterns in specific language impaired children, including semantic–pragmatic disorder, and in receptive language of age matched normal children. MSc thesis: Institute of Neurology, University of London, 1993.

Wiig E. Test of Language Competence. London: The Psychological Corporation, 1988.

Wing L. Asperger's syndrome: a clinical account. Journal of Psychological Medicine 1981; 11: 115–29.

Wing L. The continuum of autistic characteristics. In Schopler E, Mesibov GB (eds) Diagnosis and Assessment in Autism. New York: Plenum, 1988.

Wing L, Gould J. Severe impairments of social interaction and associated abnormalities in children: epidemiology and classification. Journal of Autism and Developmental Disorders 1979; 9: 1.

Chapter 4
Language-based education for children with special needs

WENDY RINALDI

Introduction

The aim of this chapter is to describe in some detail a language-based approach to teaching children with special needs and to show how this approach can facilitate more effective teaching in a range of curriculum subjects. The starting point is to explain the rationale, then to take a fairly brief look at assessment before presenting the teaching approach, including its application to curriculum subjects. Finally, the varying needs across the age range will be considered. Chapter 5 will then focus on how a language-based approach can be implemented in a special school or mainstream setting.

The term *language impaired children* is used to apply to all children with language difficulties, including children who have specific difficulties with language (including pragmatic disorder) and children whose language difficulties form part of a broader picture of special needs.

Incidental and language-based approaches

Naturalistic approaches to language intervention are based on the assumption that children will learn language best in situations where it is being used to serve communicative purposes and where it is clearly integrated into real life activities. At the heart of this approach is the assumption that children's language problems can be resolved through incidental learning. The role of the teacher or therapist is not to focus on language explicitly, but to facilitate incidental learning of language by providing appropriate linguistic input and opportunities for the child to use language (Donaldson, 1995).

This concept is one that most would want to take on board in teaching practice. However, experience shows that language impaired children cannot learn language incidentally. Rather, it is necessary first to explicitly teach particular language skills and strategies. This 'explicit teaching' enables children to use these skills/strategies in the communicative and learning opportunities which can then be created as in a naturalistic approach. Hence language teaching becomes a base or foundation for broader learning.

There is consistent research evidence of the effectiveness of explicit language teaching. For example, in a review of intervention research, Moats and Lyons (1996) conclude:

> Intervention research clearly demonstrates that individuals who are taught language explicitly progress more readily than those who are not. Given the consistency of research findings, the paucity of teachers skilled in teaching language explicitly ... is of more concern than ever (p. 73).

In the following paragraphs, the rationale for a language-based approach, as distinct from an incidental approach, is illustrated with three examples relating to curriculum subjects: Food technology, History and Mathematics.

Example 1: A lesson in Food technology

Food technology is an area of the curriculum that may be defined as 'rich in language stimulation'. An incidental approach would suggest that given an appropriate linguistic input, children would acquire the range of vocabulary associated with this subject including, for example, food types and categories, cooking methods and utensils, nutrition, hygiene and so on. However, it is important to consider the other requirements of a lesson in Food technology: the fine motor skills to carry out cooking techniques (from basic skills such as mixing/chopping to the more complex tasks, for example, of pastry making); the organizational skills to carry out cooking sequences; the ability to read or memorize recipes. These areas are commonly problematic for language impaired children. Given this level of skill demand, it can be envisaged that the children will be unlikely to give sufficient attention to language, even if the input is appropriate in terms of language levels. A language-based approach first teaches the vocabulary and concepts associated with Food technology to enable the child to make use of this learning in the practical activity and to focus on the other demands of the tasks.

Example 2: History and the concept of time

Similarly, considering the concept of time and associated vocabulary, an incidental approach would take the view that children can gain an under-standing of time by learning about History. However, language impaired children often struggle with the concept of time on a day-to-day basis; even children who are able to tell the time may not understand the underlying concept. Given other demands of History, such as historical dates and specialized vocabulary concerning historic periods (clothing, weapons, foods, etc.), which may no longer be in use, the expectations of incidental learning have unfortunately proved unrealistic. In contrast, a language-based approach concentrates on the vocabulary and conceptual associates which enable children to understand and use time concepts. They are then able to learn more effectively from the broader learning context of a History lesson.

Example 3: Measurement tasks in Mathematics

An incidental approach assumes that children will gain an appreciation of size through measurement. Early measurement tasks may be more concrete and experiential, leading to activities involving rulers/numeracy. Language impaired children, however, appear not to be able to gain an understanding of size in this way. In a sample of ten children with specific developmental language disorder (SDLD), nine were able to report that rulers were used to measure. However, when asked, using closure techniques, *what* rulers measured ('OK. So you can measure a table – and what are you measuring about the table – you're measuring its ———'), only one child was able to answer 'size'. These children thus did not have a full understanding of measurement; in particular, the purpose of measuring.

The language associated with size dimensions can also be a source of confusion to language impaired children. They can show difficulty distinguishing between height, length and width, and the varied associated vocabulary: for example, when it is appropriate to use 'fat' as opposed to 'wide'; 'tall' instead of 'high'. Language impaired children also need to be shown that the word 'short' may be used to refer to either the length or height dimension. Further, the author has found that children need to understand the concept of comparative or graded sizes to fully appreciate the relationship between units of measurement (Rinaldi, 1998).

Therefore, in a language-based approach, the concepts and vocabulary of size dimension and comparison are explicitly taught first: this learning is then applied to measurement tasks. This enables children to fully understand the mechanics of measurement and to generalize these principles to other learning situations. Similarly, the concepts/vocabulary of mass and volume are taught prior to children completing related measurement tasks.

Assessment

It is very easy to fall into the trap of assuming that language impaired children know more than they actually do. The children may have sufficient compensatory skills to complete activities without understanding the underlying learning point. In this way they can 'go through the motions' of a lesson without, in fact, learning from it. Appropriate assessment enables the teacher or therapist to identify gaps in knowledge which otherwise may remain undetected, particularly if they concern comprehension (Ehren and Lenz, 1989).

Standardized tests have value when it comes to comparing the child's language or cognitive abilities to children of similar ages. However, criterion-referenced assessments tend to give a fuller, more comprehensive picture of a child's abilities/skills than standardized tests, in particular areas of language or learning and, therefore, are usually more helpful when it comes to planning teaching.

The idea of criterion-referenced assessment is to record the child's development in relation to his or her previous performance rather than in relation to the performance of others. This kind of assessment is, there-fore, also useful in gaining a baseline record from which to measure an individual's progress and enable the teacher or therapist to judge the effectiveness of teaching in line with teaching targets. Summary measures of progress can further be shared with individual children: the author has found the use of visual presentation valuable here, where progress is shown on a colour chart or graph.

A list of language/communication skills assessments currently in common use in the UK is included in the appendix to this chapter. This list is not exhaustive, but will give the reader a starting point from which to investigate further. Some university libraries (for example, the Department of Human Communication, University College, London) give practitioners the opportunity to view a range of assessments.

Teaching overview: Key elements of a language-based approach

Deciding upon a framework: the concept of cumulative learning

The relationship between language and learning difficulties was highlighted in Chapter 1. Two elements of cognitive deficit proposed to occur in developmental language disorder were the ability to: a) process and integrate information and b) plan and organize learning.

It may be for these reasons that language impaired children appear to learn most effectively when teaching is structured to: a) break down learning into relatively small steps; b) make explicit the links between learning steps; and c) introduce new elements in a way which reinforces and adds to previous learning.

The first stage of any teaching plan therefore needs to concentrate on the development of a framework, with a clear start and end point, into which activities can be allocated in a way that will allow learning to build. Clearly, activities need to be of interest to the children and presented in a format/at a level that will enable them to access learning. However, this alone will not be sufficient: it is the way activities are **ordered** which enables children to gain a full understanding and to retain learning.

One such framework, built upon the metacognitive approach, is described later in this chapter.

Multisensory methods

In Chapters 1 and 2, deficits in auditory processing and recall were identified as a feature of language disorder. For language impaired children the auditory input channel is therefore the weakest one when it comes to learning. This makes it necessary to supplement auditory presentations in teaching/therapy with visual and kinaesthetic/experiential techniques to enable children to access and retain learning.

Experiential techniques facilitate learning for all children, in part because they enable them to become active participants in the learning process, which is generally a more motivating experience. Further, visual and experiential techniques are invaluable in increasing the salience or 'tangibility' of abstract concepts. Even concepts or skills normally acquired early on in communication development can be abstract in nature. An example here is the concept/skill of listening. The expectation is that young children will develop the process of listening for learning, perhaps with some reminders: 'Are you listening?', 'Don't forget to listen', 'Are your ears awake?', to mention but a few. Yet the concept of listening is actually abstract in nature. Children may have some sense that listening is something they should do because their teacher says so, but they may not know actually what to do. 'Listening' can therefore be broken down into particular skills or strategies which can be demonstrated. For example, a fundamental skill of listening for learning is to 'think about the same thing as the speaker'. Figure 4.1 demonstrates a visual representation of this notion. A basic listening strategy for young children is 'good sitting': *feet on floor, hands on lap, bottom back in seat*. This can easily be demonstrated and may be used to replace distracting movements such as chair rocking and excessive fidgeting.

Action and visual methods also help children to remember sequence strings. Examples of activities relating to Science and Maths sequences are referred to later in this chapter.

Procedure

In a language-based approach there are three main steps to developing a teaching plan. **The first step** is to decide upon the language/communication

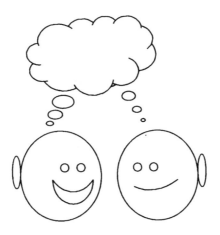

Figure 4.1 Visual representation of listening skill: *Think about the same thing as the person speaking.*

skill to be taught; for example: Which interaction skill? Which vocabulary set? Which grammatical marker? Which pragmatic skill? Which phonemic contrast? This decision will be informed by the children's learning or social needs; normal developmental patterns of language may also be considered.

The second step, which may actually inform the first, is to look at the learning and/or social impact and decide upon the subject area within which the language/communication skill can best be taught. For example, an initial decision may have been taken to develop a child's conceptual and vocabulary knowledge/use and to improve word finding abilities. Vocabulary sets can be taught in a way that will enable children to access curriculum programmes of study in particular subject areas (Science, Mathematics, Humanities, etc.). Teaching may involve establishing links between new vocabulary concepts and those that the child already knows. Alternatively, it may be necessary to develop basic vocabulary/concepts, assumed by the programme of study, to enable children to achieve broader learning targets. The initial focus will be on language (e.g. size dimensions vocabulary), but this will need to contribute to the broader learning context of a curriculum subject (in the case of size dimension, Mathematics) or social experience, if it is to be of any real value to the child. The impact of language/communication skills on curriculum subjects is dealt with in greater detail later in this chapter.

In Chapter 5 it will be suggested that different professional groups may have different starting points in educating language impaired children. For example, speech and language therapists' starting points may be with the language/communication difficulty; teachers' starting points may be with the curriculum. Therefore, speech and language therapists may start with step 1; teachers may actually start with step 2. However, this does not create a problem because, whichever is the starting point, there will be movement backward and forward between the two steps to determine teaching/therapy targets. That is, the language/communication skill to be taught is determined by the child's learning needs and the subject is taught in a way that teaches basic language knowledge to enable broader learning targets. Therefore, if the subject is the starting point (step 2) there will need to be a consideration as to which language/communication skill is to be taught (step 1) to access that subject. If the language/communication skill is the starting point (step 1) there will need to be consideration of which subject area it contributes to (step 2).

The third step is to develop a series of activities, with a build-up to learning, starting with comprehension and progressing to use. One such activity sequence, based on a metacognitive approach, is described on page 86.

Steps 1 and 2: The impact of a language focus on curriculum subjects

Effects across the curriculum

The 'going in and staying in' factor

The principles underpinning the language-based approach described in this chapter serve to give children access to education across the curriculum and to retain learning. A multisensory methodology is one key to access; another is the avoidance of learning overload and the planning of teaching/therapy to enable children to make links between new knowledge and skills and what they already know. Multisensory methods also contribute to the 'staying in' factor because children are more likely to remember visualization or direct experience of particular learning points. The organization of teaching/therapy to allow cumulative learning is also important here because this provides reinforcement of key learning points.

Demonstrating learning

A technique commonly used by teachers to monitor the effectiveness of teaching is to ask children to demonstrate their learning through oral or written communication. The language skills required here concern a) the concepts and vocabulary relating to subject areas and b) the ability to select and organize information adequately from the array of possible alternatives. In Chapter 3 it was noted that some children have such difficulty with selection and organizational language skills that they cannot offer any response. Without these skills it is quite possible that children who do actually learn within a subject area will nevertheless fail to demonstrate this learning adequately. The ability to select and organize language can be taught as part of the English curriculum, as demonstrated in the following section.

English

An area of language chiefly concerned in English is that of pragmatics. Phonology inputs substantially to literacy. Grammatical skills can affect the clarity of spoken language and the accuracy of written language. The semantic area is concerned in extending vocabulary.

Pragmatics

Pragmatics was described in some depth in Chapter 3. In summary, pragmatics was conceptualized as comprising three key elements:

- The interactive process of communication.
- The selection and organization of language appropriate to listener need. This aspect of pragmatics incorporates the notion of relevance and sufficiency.
- The comprehension of meaning open to interpretation.

It is with reference to these elements that English will now be considered.

Pragmatics and the English curriculum

Building on their previous experience, children should be encouraged to speak with confidence, making themselves clear through *organising what they say and choosing words with precision.* They should be taught to incorporate *relevant detail in explanations, descriptions and narratives,* and to *distinguish between the essential and the less important, taking into account the needs of their listeners.* Pupils should be taught *conventions of discussion and conversation,* e.g. taking turns in conversation, and how to *structure their talk in ways that are coherent* and understandable (Department of Education, 1995).

The above quotation clearly demonstrates the relation between pragmatic skills and English.

There are a number of teaching resources available which focus specifically on conversational skills (Rustin and Khur, 1989; Rinaldi, 1992, 1995; Kelly, 1996).

The ability to organize language and to distinguish what is important from what is non-essential in relation to listener need, can be taught through a metacognitive approach (Rinaldi, 1999). This involves a breakdown of teaching targets as outlined in Figure 4.2.

A further pragmatic skill required for English is that of contextual understanding; in particular the interplay between context and word or sentence meaning. The ability to make interpretations inferred by contextual

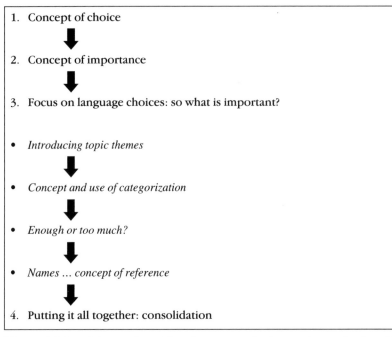

1. Concept of choice

2. Concept of importance

3. Focus on language choices: so what is important?

- *Introducing topic themes*

- *Concept and use of categorization*

- *Enough or too much?*

- *Names ... concept of reference*

4. Putting it all together: consolidation

Figure 4.2 Breakdown of teaching: language selection and organization. Taken from Rinaldi (1999).

information may be needed to follow spoken discussions and written texts. In Chapter 3 it was shown how many words and phrases carry multiple meanings: the decision as to which meaning is intended can be derived through contextual understanding. A further illustration is included in Figure 4.3.

The idea of context contributing to meaning is one that may need to be explicitly taught to language impaired children. The author has found that this can be achieved through visual analogy and role-play exercises (Rinaldi, 1996).

Utterance: 'Jenny, you need to pull your socks up'

Context implying literal interpretation appropriate: Jenny is wearing socks which are around her ankles

Context implying idiomatic interpretation appropriate: The utterance is made in connection with a piece of work/behaviour which needs improving. Jenny's socks (if she is wearing any) do not need pulling up

---

Figure 4.3 Example to illustrate the use of context to determine intended meaning.

Grammatical skills and English

Language impaired children may make errors of syntax or morphology in grammar. Syntactic errors concern disruption to the construction of words into phrases (The tabby cat), phrases into sentences (The tabby cat [phrase 1] was eating [phrase 2]), and sentence combinations (The tabby cat was eating [sentence 1] *because* [relation] he was hungry [sentence 2]). Children may make omissions or order errors (e.g. 'the cat tabby' instead of 'the tabby cat'; 'eating the cat' instead of 'the cat eating', etc.).

Morphological errors of grammar concern grammatical markers which carry meaning such as plural 's' (signals 'more than one'), possessive 's' (signals belonging) and tense markers (signals past, present or future). Children may omit markers or use them incorrectly.

Some grammatical errors, for example, omission of third person singular (the girl like her new trousers) or omission of determiner 'the' in noun phrases (man went home; I saw girl laughing) create inaccuracies in written work and sound immature in spoken language. Other errors also affect accuracy of meaning, as shown in the cat eating example above.

These aspects of grammatical ability appear particularly resistant to development; errors may persist if they are not addressed specifically. For example, in a group of 15 teenagers with language impairments and moderate learning difficulties, five continued to have difficulty in marking pronouns appropriately; seven had difficulty marking tense (Rinaldi, 1992). The activities listed later in the chapter can be used to develop grammatical skills.

Phonology and literacy

Children with phonological difficulties may omit or substitute phonemes or phonemic blends in a way that affects their speech intelligibility. There may also be difficulties with syllable structure in multi-syllabic words.

By the time children enter school some of their phonological difficulties may have resolved, either spontaneously or through intervention. However, underlying difficulties may persist: the metaphonological skills relating to an awareness of the use of sound, sound patterns and syllable structure, self-monitoring abilities and so on. These kind of skills need to be developed to establish appropriate phonology in spoken language and can also be extended to phoneme–grapheme (sound–letter) correspondence in developing skills of literacy. A number of studies have shown that this kind of work impacts on reading and spelling abilities (Cunningham, 1990; Ball and Blachman, 1991; Byrne and Fielding Barnsley 1993, Popple and Wellington, 1996). Popple and Wellington present two case studies where working on phonological processing assisted reading and spelling abilities. In a collaborative approach, skills developed included discrimination and production of sounds and phoneme–grapheme correspondence, syllable segmentation and semantic/phonemic cueing to facilitate word finding.

Semantic elements: developing vocabulary for English

In English, children are required to use language descriptively and to explore and develop ideas with increasing complexity as they grow older. Children with language impairments may continue to use a basic, simplified vocabulary set unless they are specifically helped to extend their vocabulary. For some children this will occur as a result of word-finding difficulties: 'vague' vocabulary, such as 'get', 'do', 'go' to represent verbs or 'stuff', 'thing' to represent nouns, may be the only type of vocabulary they can access at the time of communication. The author has also found that much of language impaired children's talk at primary and secondary school is descriptive in nature: children very rarely talk about their opinions or thoughts. Children's vocabulary can be extended in these areas by using links with vocabulary that they already know, by way of the brainstorm technique (section entitled 'Brainstorming' later in this chapter). Linking words in this way can also alleviate word-finding difficulties. An example, relating to the word 'good', is included in Figure 4.4.

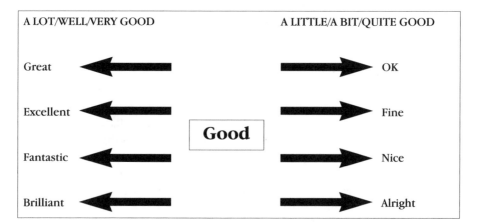

Figure 4.4 Brainstorming to extend vocabulary knowledge. Example: good.

Mathematics

The area of language of most relevance in Mathematics is semantics, in particular, the understanding and use of language concepts and associated vocabulary. Language concepts needed for Maths include shape; pattern; size and measurement; quantity and number; calculation; fraction; time;

probability, chance and prediction. Knowledge of these concepts is vital if children are to follow Maths programmes of study, for example, those included in National Curriculum (England and Wales) attainment targets: Handling Data; Shape, Space and Measure and Applying Mathematics.

Science

The area of semantics, in particular that of conceptual/vocabulary under-standing and use, is also crucial in enabling children to access Science. There is a wealth of vocabulary to be learned, for example, in relation to life processes and living things (human body parts and processes; animal groups; plant processes) materials and properties (recognizing common materials; changes to states of matter, density, colour/shade, etc.) and physical processes (forces, electricity, gravity, etc.).

Scientific concepts such as density, gravity, photosynthesis and digestion, to name but a few, can prove difficult for language impaired children to understand because of their abstract nature. Language can actually be used as a vehicle to enable children to grasp these concepts because links can be 'chained back' to those concepts/vocabulary with which the children are already familiar. For example, in work focusing on recognizing common materials, **CHINA** can be associated with, 'hard'; 'can break when you drop it' and 'opaque'; as distinct from **GLASS**, which is 'hard', 'can break' but is (usually) 'transparent' and **METAL**, which is 'hard', 'does not break when you drop it', and is opaque. 'Transparent' can be further linked to 'you can see through it', 'opaque' to 'you can't see through it'. 'Hard' can be further associated with description (and action), e.g. 'you can knock on it'; 'you can't squeeze it'. Other examples are included in Rinaldi (1998).

Geography and History

As in the case of Science and Mathematics, it is the understanding of concepts and vocabulary associates which enables access to the more detailed study of Geography and History.

As in all subjects, skills of organizational language, grammar and phonology are needed to express learning in both the written and the spoken modalities.

In Geography, children are required to study particular countries in detail, interpret and make maps and globes, appreciate geographical context and use appropriate geographical vocabulary. The author's experience suggests that assessment of language impaired children at key stage 2 (7–11 years) can reveal, however, that they may lack understanding of even fundamental concepts relating to these areas of study. For example, knowledge gaps were identified with regard to the concept of mapping (What is a map? Why do we use maps?), geographical structure of countries (for example, the arrangement of villages and towns in relation to cities), and the relationship between countries and continents. Furthermore, language impaired children can develop a very narrow style of conceptualization. For example, in studying weather types with a group of 10-year-old SDLD children the author discovered that all associated 'rain' with cold temperatures only and 'sun' with hot temperatures only.

A key language concept to gain access to History concerns an element of the time concept: an appreciation of past in relation to present. This can be taught using time lines, starting with the present day ('now') and moving back in time. An effective method here is to focus on one aspect of living (for example, clothing, eating, housing, transport) to show how it changed from the present day. Links can then be made moving forward in time to the present day, showing changes in relation to modernization, invention, legislation, etc. Using distinct categories such as 'war time', 'Victorians (Queen Victoria)'; 'Tudors'; 'Anglo Saxons', also helps children to conceptualize the sequence of changes over time.

History can also present difficulties for language impaired children because a fair amount of the vocabulary included (for example with reference to clothing, transport, weapons, law and order) is no longer in current use and thus harder to remember. The students are more likely to be able to remember this vocabulary if links are made to the present.

'Non-academic' subjects: PE, Art and Music

PE, Art and Music are commonly regarded as subjects where language impaired children can do well, because there are minimum requirements of language. Certainly, at a practical level, language impaired children can develop an appreciation of these subjects and do very well indeed, without understanding the related language concepts. However, language concepts do clearly play a part in these subject areas. In PE, for example, children may need to follow instructions requiring an understanding of spatial concepts/vocabulary, such as 'forward, backward, left/right, over/under', etc.

Musical tasks may require children to follow instructions including vocabulary relating to concepts of volume, speed, pitch, etc. Art activities may include instructions that require comprehension of concepts/vocabulary such as colour, shade, texture and spatial awareness.

Personal and social education

Children need effective interactive communication skills to do well socially, and more so as they grow older. At this time social relationships rely increasingly upon communication skills: notes, chat, jokes and so on. Children who have difficulties with interactive communication may fail to give listener feedback through, for example, eye contact, appropriate questioning or facial expression, and thus appear uninterested in peers. Others who disregard turn-taking and other conversational rules may appear to 'hog' the conversation and seem egocentric.

Further, in order to become independent young people, children need to be able to deal effectively with a range of social contexts, such as ordering food in public eating places, seeking information about public transport, returning faulty goods to shops, making health appointments etc. Poor interactive skills place students at a disadvantage here. For example, the author has observed that children with communication difficulties can fail to signal their wish to communicate by engaging in eye contact. In a busy shop queue scenario this can result in them not getting served.

Interviews with language impaired children have revealed that they can lack self awareness and may be unaware of even basic friendship strategies. Language can provide a vehicle, through category sets, to focus students' thinking on their interests (for example, sport, films, books, careers, special interests, etc.) and on how knowledge of shared interests can be used to develop friendship. There may also be a need to focus teaching explicitly on how students can appropriately express their feelings, and recognize the feelings of others, both through words and non-verbal communication (facial expression, body movement/posture and tone of voice). There may further be a need to familiarize students with vocabulary and phrases to be able to express their opinions and to seek the opinions of others. The activity described in Figure 4.5 focuses on this area.

In Chapter 1, it was noted that children with special needs might be prone to poor self esteem. There are a number of procedures that may be incorporated into a broader teaching philosophy/style to develop

---

Activity: I think....What do you think?

The activity leader shows the students the following food menu[1]

        Cheesy eggs

        Liver and bacon in chocolate sauce

        Coffee cake and ice cream

Each student is invited to say one opinion about the menu (for example about a like/dislike, nutritional content, vegetarian issue, etc.), using the words *I think*....They then ask someone else in the group to say their opinion using the words *What do you think....(name of person)*. In this way, ideas bounce across the circle and the students are able to hear and use appropriate vocabulary/phrases.

Figure 4.5 Activity to develop expression opinion/seeking opinion of others. Taken from Social Use of Language Programme, Rinaldi (revised edition in progress).

---

[1] Other examples include fashion designs, tape of different music excerpts, a selection of competition prizes, etc.

children's self-concept and to prevent self esteem spiralling downward (for example, Rogers, 1994, 1998; Beattie, 1996). The author has found that it is important to view failure as a positive, inevitable process in children's learning. This can be demonstrated, for example, by praising children when they make mistakes with statements such as 'well done, you're learning'. This kind of feedback enables children to more confidently attempt to put the mistake right, or to accept help in putting it right. Group activities and story material (see for example Rinaldi, 1995, 1997) can also be used to increase children's awareness of their strengths and the acceptability of having weaknesses, many of which can be improved.

Figure 4.6 summarizes the relation between areas of language/communication and curriculum subjects. In the following section a method to teach language/communication skills to children with special needs, integral to curriculum subjects, is presented.

	ENGLISH	MATHS/ SCIENCE	HUMANITIES	PSE
Phonology	**X** (literacy)	X	X	X
Grammar	**X**	X	X	X
Semantic elements: concept knowledge, categorization etc.	X	**X**	**X**	**X**
Pragmatics • Interaction • Relevance/ Sufficiency • Inference	**X**	X	X	**X**

Figure 4.6 Aspects of language/communication in relation to curriculum subjects. Bold **X** indicates where language areas chiefly contribute.

Step 3: Developing a cumulative activity sequence: a metacognitive approach

Overview

The central philosophy of a metacognitive approach is that the student (child or adult) becomes aware of the learning process itself in addition to the actual content of learning.

Therefore, a key element is: awareness (or comprehension) before use. That is, students cannot be expected to meaningfully use or generalize a point of learning unless they fully understand it and appreciate its purpose.

Metacognitive approaches have been incorporated into teaching/ therapy to develop behaviour (Rogers, 1994, 1998), memory and study skills (Mitchell, 1998). In the area of language and communication, metacognitive approaches have been applied to phonology (Dean and Howell, 1990), grammar (Rinaldi, in press), semantics (Rinaldi, 1998) and pragmatics (Rinaldi 1992, 1995, 1997, 1999).

The activity sequence listed in this section is one that has been developed by the author to apply the metacognitive approach to the area of language/communication development. An overview is included in Figure 4.7. Subsequent paragraphs explain the principles underpinning the development of these activities, with some illustration of application to the different language areas. Particular examples are drawn from the author's own work and the reader will also be able to consider other resources (published and 'home-made') within this framework. On reading these paragraphs it will be useful to keep in mind the ways in which the different language areas will impact upon curriculum subjects and social times, as discussed earlier in this chapter.

In Figure 4.7, a number of activities have been listed in the 'awareness' and 'use' sections. It is not always necessary to complete all of these

1. **Awareness activities: Enabling children to understand the 'whats and whys'**
- Stories
- Drama sketches
- Posters
- Deliberate mistakes
- Communication models
- Problem solving
- Visual analogies
- Brainstorms
- Hiding/matching games
- Action sequences

2. **Practice activities: Enabling children to achieve the 'what and how'**
- Game activities
- Talking practice
- Acted scenarios
- Carryover tasks

Figure 4.7 Metacognitive approach: overview and activity sequence.

activities, but some students require a good deal of reinforcement to learn. Further, certain activities lend themselves more readily than others to particular areas of language and so it is useful to become familiar with the variety of activity types listed.

The examples in the following section relate to a number of different language areas (semantics, grammar, pragmatics, etc.). *It is important to note, however, that the activity sequence is applied separately to each aspect of language being taught (for example, a phonemic contrast or a vocabulary set or a grammatical marker or an interactive communication skill) within each subject. Attempting to cover a number of language areas simultaneously, that is, within the same activity or activity sequence, is likely to cause 'learning overload'.* This point is clarified by the examples in Figure 4.16 on page 100. The reader may like to refer to this figure before reading the activity descriptions.

In summary, the procedure starts by selecting a language skill/concept (for example, a phonemic contrast, a vocabulary set, a grammatical marker, an interactive communication skill) which will enable access to a curriculum subject (or aspect of social development). The language skill/concept is then taught through the activity sequence: at the end of the sequence the skill is applied to a broader learning or social experience. When children have mastered and applied this skill, the next is selected for that subject, and so the process continues.

Activities: rationale and illustration

Awareness/comprehension

Developing stories. The author has developed a series of steps to create story lines which have proved effective for children with special needs, as a starting point to initiate progress. These steps are listed in Figure 4.8.

Stories incorporating the above steps are used to help children to become more aware of their errors, so that they can replace them with appropriate strategies.

The stories have also been useful in helping children to see the outcomes of their actions (steps 3 and 4) and to appreciate why it is important to change – from their viewpoint and from the viewpoint of others. This has proved a helpful process to children across special needs groups, perhaps most interestingly including children with autism, who may have impaired 'Theory of Mind' (this kind of impairment is described in Chapter 3).

At first thought, it may appear to the teacher or therapist that making the child more aware of his/her difficulties/errors may be a very negative and perhaps unproductive exercise. In fact, children with special needs do usually have some sense that they are 'getting things wrong', no matter

1. Choose a character children can relate to and enjoy

2. Show character having same problem as child (e.g. a grammatical error **or** inappropriate use of a vocabulary set **or** poor eye contact/ listening skills)[2]

3. Show effect on others (e.g. other characters are confused or upset)

4. Show effect back on character (e.g. other characters don't understand/don't want to be friends)

5. Introduce strategies to alleviate problem (e.g. correct grammatical expression or correct vocabulary or appropriate eye contact/listening skills)

6. Show positive outcome

7. Include talking points at the end of the story to focus on key learning points and to enable the students to relate to the characters

Figure 4.8 Steps in developing story lines.

how hard those who care for or teach them try to protect them from this discovery. However, a metacognitive approach gives children a much fuller and more positive understanding of why they are having a particular difficulty and, very importantly, gives them a means of moving on. There is also a great sense of achievement to be gained by knowing that you have moved on, which can't be experienced if you didn't know you were getting things wrong in the first place! It is for these reasons that the metacognitive approach has been associated with children having a greater 'control' or sense of their own learning and, perhaps, accounts in some way for anecdotal evidence (parental/teacher reports) of improved self esteem seen in children who are taught using this approach.

The use of characters which the students can relate to and enjoy is a very important 'ingredient' in developing stories, because despite the points made in the previous paragraph, enabling children to gain a fuller insight into their difficulties (in order to progress) is a sensitive area. The use of characters enables the children to observe and make comments from a 'third-person viewpoint' which is always easier than attempting to directly view one's own behaviour or skills. The talking points at the end of the story (for example: Do you have problems like —— (the character)? How can you make things better?), then enables children to look at their

---

[2] Only *one* communication error should be selected, e.g. failure to mark plural (grammar) **or** incorrect use/gaps in knowledge relating to one vocabulary set (semantics) e.g. size or shape, etc.

own behaviour or communication. The author has found that children are far more willing to look at their own difficulties when they have seen a character, which they enjoyed reading about, having the same problems.

The author has successfully used characters and story lines to develop interactive skills of communication (Rinaldi, 1995, 1997) and grammar (Rinaldi, in press). Work currently being developed has also included story material to develop concepts/vocabulary of colour (for example, Roger Red would only eat tomatoes), shape (The Shape Family) and size (The Size Magician). The story line used to develop eye contact in the *Looking Luke Story* (Rinaldi, 1995) is outlined in Figure 4.9.

1/2. Luke has a problem with eye contact. His friend, Moby, tries to talk to him – but Luke looks at the flowers ... the trees ... birds ... not at Moby
3.   Moby is upset – he wants Luke to look at him – he wants to be friends
4.   Luke is sad – he wants to be friends with Moby and he has made him cross
5.   Moby tells Luke: look at me when we talk
6.   Luke looks at Moby and Moby looks at Luke ... they talk about lots of different things – they are very good friends
7.   Talking points: Do you have problems like Luke? What can you do?

Figure 4.9 Story line: *Looking Luke Story*; Social Use of Language Programme Infant/Primary School (Rinaldi, 1995).

When the underlying principles are understood, the use of story material offers an extremely versatile teaching method, which can be incorporated as a first step to develop communicative, learning or behavioural strategies. Using the guidelines summarised in Figure 4.8, the possibilities are endless!

Drama sketches. As an alternative or an addition to stories, staff can act out story lines (live or on video) taking the role of the story characters. Alternatively, puppets or toys can be used. This can be a more effective presentation for children with visual impairments or for young children who have difficulty interpreting two-dimensional representations. It is important, as with the stories, that the children are observers here. As with the stories, the students' thinking should be focused on the key learning points either during the sketch (via freeze frames) or at the end of it, with simple questions such as: *What went wrong? What can —— do?*

Posters. The key learning points of the stories can be visually reinforced by poster material. An advantage of posters is that they can be used in many different settings at school and home. They can therefore be used to show children how they can use particular strategies in a variety of different contexts. 'Pop-up' picture displays can be developed for younger children.

Hiding and matching games. These kinds of activities are useful for teaching new words to young (and not so young) children. It is now fairly well documented (for example, Crystal, 1987; Rinaldi, 1998) that children learn and retain vocabulary most effectively if they are taught in groups or categories. In this way, the children are being given a strategy for storing and retrieving words in addition to expanding their knowledge of word meanings. Matching items (pictured or real) to their group or category words provides one way of introducing this strategy to young children, and, essentially in a metacognitive approach, the idea of words 'going together in groups' with a 'group name' is specifically taught as part of this activity. An extension of the activity is to ask children to find hidden items (pictured or real) associated with particular categories: each child, or pair of children, is given a different category to find. Specific examples relating to concepts for Mathematics, Science and Geography are included in Rinaldi (1998).

Visual analogies. It is sometimes possible to develop a visual analogy to represent an abstract concept. This serves to increase the salience of the concept and can give children access to learning points that would other-wise be too obscure to grasp.

An example to illustrate here is the notion of introducing topics and topic shifts. In Chapter 3 it was noted that language impaired children can sometimes fail to appreciate the importance of 'signposting' their talk; they can show a tendency to launch into specific details and switch topics without alerting the listener. The author has found that children need to appreciate the distinction between 'outline' and 'detail' to enable them to apply the concept of topic introduction and shift to their talk. Children can access the distinction between 'outline' (or 'sketch') and 'detail' through an analogy with drawing. The activity outlined in Figure 4.10 (taken from Rinaldi, 1999) has proved useful here, for both junior and secondary school-aged students.

Action sequences. Action sequences to incorporate visual and experiential learning are particularly useful in helping children to remember sequence strings, in addition to understanding relevant vocabulary. For example, children may be asked to walk the digestive system, act out an electricity sequence, walk 'the day' (Rinaldi, 1998) and so on.

Deliberate mistakes. These activities are useful to check and consolidate children's language comprehension. They can be used with children of all ages. The activity leader simply makes deliberate mistakes that the

PREPARATION: You will need some A1 sheets of paper or you can use a white/black-board.

DOING THE ACTIVITY: The activity leader instructs the students that they have to guess what he/she is drawing. The activity leader then draws a house, but **starting with small details** – for example, drawing the bricks, windowsills, etc. The picture should be drawn so that it will take a while for the students to guess what it is. The activity leader times how long it takes for the students to guess correctly and tells them afterwards. The activity leader then starts a second picture, asking the students to guess as soon as they know what it's about. **This time the activity leader should draw a house outline** – the students should be able to guess almost immediately. The activity leader then summarizes the main learning points and links to communication. For example: *OK so both my pictures were about a house – the first time (show picture) I started with something we call **detail** – all the **little bits** of the house like the bricks and windowsills – it took you a long time to know what my picture was about. But then I drew the shape of the house – we call this the **outline** – and you knew what my picture was about straight away. Well, it's like that with talking. If you go into all the little **details** (show first picture) the person doesn't know what you're talking about – they might get fed up listening – but if you give them the **outline** first (show second picture) then they know what you're talking about straight away – it's much more interesting.*

This activity should then be repeated with further examples, such as a leaf, a dog, a cup. The activity leader should just choose one way of drawing each of these examples, i.e. either starting with detail (veins on the leaf, fur/whiskers on the dog, pattern on the cup, etc.) **or** outline. The students then have to guess whether the activity leader gave them the **outline** or the **details**.

Figure 4.10 Visual analogy activity: introducing topics. Taken from Language Choices (Rinaldi, 1999).

children need to identify. The activity can be formalized into a game called 'Right or Wrong?' (or 'Yes or No?'), where the activity leader attempts to correctly use, for example, a word, a grammatical marker, a non-verbal communication skill, or a speech sound, etc., – depending upon which aspect of language is being focused upon. The children, in turn, say whether the leader is right or wrong.

The idea of making deliberate errors is extended further in the communication/behaviour models described in the following section.

Communication/behaviour models. The communication/behaviour models require two members of staff to show inappropriate and then appropriate use of a behaviour or communication skill. Models can be shown 'live' to the students or on a video. One of the staff members starts by demonstrating poor use of a communication/language skill or an inappropriate behaviour (referred to as 'mirroring' by Rogers, 1998), demonstrating the kinds of errors the students make; the other member of staff uses appropriate skills. It is important to focus on one communication skill or one kind of behaviour at any one time. The errors are made fairly obvious to enable the students to easily observe them. The model should last about 30 seconds.

The communication partner's response is as important as the person modelling the poor communication skills/behaviour: they should become obviously upset. This enables students to see the outcome of making the error and identifies reasons to improve on the skill or change the behaviour. These lines of thinking are brought out in a series of questions which are put to the children after the model, as follows:

- Was that OK?
- What was wrong?
- How do you think———— (communication partner) felt?

The activity leader then asks the staff member playing the communication partner:

- What was it like talking to me? (partner replies how they felt: uncomfortable, irritated, etc.)
- How about friendship? Would that be OK? (or to younger children: can we be friends?) (partner replies: no way!)

The activity leader finishes feedback discussion by asking students:

- What can I do to improve?

The staff then both demonstrate appropriate use of skills (again, about 30 seconds) and follow this up with the same feedback questions, as outlined above.

Experience has shown that staff usually need to practise the models before showing them to the children. The models will be more effective if each member of staff knows more or less what they (and each other) will say. An example script to demonstrate poor and appropriate listening skills is outlined in Figure 4.11. Other communication skills that can be modelled in this way include sufficiency and relevance of information (Rinaldi, 1999), interpretation of inferred meaning (Rinaldi, 1996), speed/volume of talking and conversational turn-taking ('interruption' versus appropriate timing, or 'hogging the conversation' versus 'sharing talking') (Rinaldi 1992, 1995).

Take 1

Speaker (staff member A): Did you hear about Mrs Smith's holiday?

Listener (staff member B) [looking out the window; fidgeting]: Eh?

Staff A: She had a terrible time – when she arrived at the hotel, her room had been given to someone else.

Staff B: I don't know what I'm going to have for my tea tonight.

Staff A: Oh – well, anyway that wasn't the end for poor Mrs Smith – she ended up having to stay at a camping site! – and it rained the whole time!

Staff B (still fidgeting; looking around the room): You know, this classroom really needs painting.

Staff A: ————(staff B's name) I wasn't talking about the classroom – I was telling you about Mrs Smith

Staff B: Oh, well – hey I'm going to get my hair cut this weekend.

Staff A: Oh that's nice – do you think we should buy Mrs Smith some flowers to make up for her holiday going wrong?

Staff B: Eh? What holiday?

Staff A: (sounding and looking fed up) Oh never mind.

Staff B (to students)

— Was that OK?

— What was wrong?

— How do you think ———— (communication partner) felt?

Staff B (to staff A)

— What was it like talking to me? (staff A replies how they felt: uncomfortable, irritated, etc.)

— How about friendship? Would that be OK? (staff A replies: no thanks)

The activity leader finishes feedback discussion by asking students:

— What can I do to improve? (Elicit: make eye contact/look at staff A; stop fidgeting; think about the same thing as staff A)

Take 2

Speaker (staff A): Did you hear about Mrs Smith's holiday?

Listener (staff B): No? what happened?

Staff A: She had a terrible time – when she arrived at the hotel, her room had been given to someone else.

Staff B: Oh no!

Staff A: And that wasn't the end – she ended up having to stay at a camping site! And it rained all the time!

Staff B: Oh dear camping holidays can be fun – but not if it rains all the time.

Staff A: Do you think we should buy Mrs Smith some flowers to make up for her holiday going wrong?

Staff B: Yeah – good idea!

Staff B (to students)

— Was that OK this time?

— Did I look at ——— (staff A)? Did I fidget? Did I think about the same thing as him/her?

— How do you think ———— (communication partner) felt this time?

Staff B (to staff A)

— What was it like talking to me? (staff A replies how they felt: much better, you were interested, etc.)

— How about friendship? Would that be OK? (staff A replies: yes, fine)

Figure 4.11 Script for a communication model: poor/appropriate listening skills.

Brainstorming. Brainstorms or "thought-sharing exercises", provide a positive way of structuring a discussion and of reviewing the learning points of previous activity (i.e. stories, communication models, etc.).

The discussion topic or idea (for example, *The 'whats' and 'whys' of listening; The 'whats' and 'whys' of taking turns; I have problems getting my words out when …*) is written (or represented pictorially) on a board or large sheet of paper so that all the children can see it. Taking turns around the circle, each child tries to contribute an idea, or repeat an idea they agree with. All ideas are written (or drawn) on the chart; even ideas which may be inaccurate. In the second stage of the brainstorm, the activity leader helps the children to identify the inaccurate ideas to take out of the brainstorm, so that only the accurate ones remain.

Social communication problem solving; modelled outcomes. The author has extended the technique of social problem solving to make it more suitable for children with special needs. It is an activity that is particularly valuable in helping junior and secondary school students to develop assertive patterns of communication and behaviour in social contexts which are commonly problematic and which may otherwise lead to aggressive behaviour or avoidance (Rinaldi, 1992, 1996; Guilford, 1988). These contexts include, for example, requests for clarification in front of peers, the use of compromise to resolve conflict with peers and family members and the ability to respond appropriately to constructive criticism.

Problem-solving activities have been used to enable children to think laterally about ways in which they can attempt to deal with these social scenarios. A problem is written up on a chart, as in a brainstorming session, and each member of the group suggests a course of action that they think will solve the problem. Example problems include: a) *My teacher keeps using words I don't understand: what can I do?* b) *I bought a pair of trainers. I spent all my birthday money on them. I had only been wearing them for one hour and the stitching came undone: what can I do?* c) *I bought a pizza in my local restaurant. When it came it wasn't the one I ordered – it had mushrooms and sweetcorn on it – I hate mushrooms and sweetcorn. I ate it, but I didn't like it much. What could I do instead if it happens again?* Other examples are included in the Social Use of Language Programme (Rinaldi, 1992).

When all the ideas for 'solving' the problem have been suggested, there follows a discussion on each suggestion, where likely outcomes of the suggestion (negative and/or positive) are identified, with a final decision being made as to whether the suggestion is likely to be helpful or not.

The author has found it necessary to adapt the discussion part of the problem in order to increase the value of the activity for students with special needs. In part, this is because children with language impairments can find discussions hard going in terms of language expression and/or comprehension, but mainly because they find it difficult to predict outcomes of their own actions and may not be swayed by the staff's interpretations. The author has found that the discussion part of the problem solve can therefore quite easily become an unproductive argument with students not appreciating the need for change.

A more effective alternative has been to *show* the students the potential outcomes of their suggestions to solve the problem in acted out scenarios. It appears that this more visual approach is more effective in enabling students to gain a more accurate perspective as to the outcomes of their actions/suggestions. As in all awareness activities, it is the members of staff who act; the students observe, reflect and comment.

The problem solve is therefore completed in three steps as summarized in Figure 4.12.

Each problem is dealt with over a minimum of two sessions

Step 1
- The problem is written up on a board/chart.
- Taking turns around the circle, each student suggests a possible 'solution' (or agrees with a 'solution' already stated).

Step 2
- After the session the staff work out simple scripts to show the students outcomes of their suggestions.
- Positive outcomes are shown for assertive behaviours; negative outcomes are shown for passive or aggressive behaviours.

Step 3
- At the next teaching session, staff model the suggested 'solutions' and outcomes.
- Students decide upon which of the solutions with a positive outcome they will practice.

Figure 4.12 Three steps of social problem solving (Rinaldi, revised Social Use of Language Programme, in progress).

Negative outcomes are shown for suggestions to solve the problem which include aggressive or passive/withdrawn behaviour. Positive outcomes are shown for assertive behaviour, but after the model staff make the point that these forms of behaviour may not always be successful: they are more likely to be successful than the other suggestions. These points are made with the aim of developing a more realistic perspective in the students. Students then practise the assertive behaviour with the staff in acted out scenarios and then in real-life contexts as described under *Talking Practice* in the next section.

It should be noted that problems can be dealt with in a series of stages of increasing difficulty. For example, in the 'trainers example' cited above, in the first stage, a positive outcome can be shown in a model where 'a student' (acted by staff member) requests a refund from a shop assistant. In this first stage the shop assistant agrees to the student's request for a refund immediately (in the model and in the subsequent talking practice). In the next stage, the problem is that the shop assistant refuses the refund. The staff then demonstrate, for example, 'staying calm' and appropriate ways to ask to see the manager.

Use: student's practice

In the following set of activities, the students are required to practise the use of a skill or behaviour that they now fully understand, having completed the awareness activities. The need for the students' practice is usually integral to the activity so that, with help from staff (as illustrated below), the students can monitor their own performance and make the necessary improvements.

Games. A variety of games can be used to develop use of language skills. For example, card games, board games and dominoes can be developed to encourage use of vocabulary or grammatical markers. Blank playing cards, available for example from a number of suppliers (or do-it-yourself stores), are invaluable for creating vocabulary/grammar card games, such as Pairs and Happy Families. Magazine photographs or drawings can be secured on one side of the cards to elicit the target vocabulary (e.g. foods; animals; transport, etc.) or grammatical markers (e.g. singular/plural; personal pronouns). An adapted version of Happy Families to focus on comprehension and use of vocabulary sets is described in Rinaldi (1998).

Group game activities can also be used to develop interactive communications skills such as eye contact, listening and turn-taking. The 'Come into my chair' activity described in Figure 4.13 has been useful for developing eye contact in children of all ages. The Go–Stop game, also described in Figure 4.13, promotes simple listening and verbal turn-taking skills.

The game activities provide a useful starting point into practice as they usually require fairly simple use of a skill in a fun format, which gives the children the confidence to tackle the more difficult forms of practice

---

Come into my chair

The activity leader stands behind a chair and makes eye contact with each student in turn (if possible the students should be sitting or standing in a line facing the chair). The students must, in turn, sit in the chair when the activity leader has made eye contact with them. The students can then each have a turn at standing behind the chair to make eye contact with one other person in the group — who then must sit in the chair.

The go–stop game

The game starts with each person in the group saying go, in turn, around the circle. The group is then told that each person can say 'stop' on two occasions. When this happens, the turns change directions. For example: Mark: go; Wendy: go; Sarah: go; Emma: go; Danny: STOP!; Emma: go; Sarah: go; Wendy: STOP! Sarah : STOP! Wendy: Go; Mark: STOP! Wendy: go; Sarah: go; Emma: STOP! Sarah: go …etc.

Figure 4.13 Examples of game activities (taken from Rinaldi, 1995).

attempted later. It is however important to ask students to identify the key learning points after each game, as there is a danger that they can become distracted by the fun elements and forget the learning purpose!

Talking practice. The students' use of language needs to extend beyond the game activities to more closely reflect everyday communicative contexts. For example, the activity described in Figure 4.14 extends the use of basic listening skills (good sitting; think about the same things as the speaker; eye contact). The use of speaking and listening seats focuses explicitly on the two-way process of communication. The 'chat-show

---

— Students are asked to practise appropriate use of skills: eye contact; appropriate sitting/ posture; thinking about the same thing as the speaker.
— Each student's turn should be no longer than 2 minutes, but may be as little as 30 seconds.
— Students practise with a member of staff. The use of a listening and speaking seat emphasizes the role of speaker and listener: each student sits in the listening seat, whilst the staff member sits in the speaking seat.
— Staff need to plan what they will speak about beforehand. It is clearly important that the content is of interest to the student practising, and to the other students in the group who will also be listening.
— Other students are involved by giving feedback to the student practising on how well they did.

Figure 4.14 Conversation practice: listening skills (taken from Rinaldi, 1992, 1995).

expert' scenario described in Figure 4.15 provides a fun format to enable children to use target vocabulary. The example given refers to food and nutritional categories, but this is an activity that can be applied to a variety of concept/vocabulary sets.

PREPARATION : You will need to video this. The students are included in the prepa-ration. They are told that they have been invited on to a chat show as food experts. The group is organized into teams of two or three people and each team is given a body needs category to be expert in, i.e. there's a team of energy (fat/carbohydrate) experts, a team of growing and mending (protein) experts and a team of 'food to help digestion' (fibre) experts. They are told that there is a million pounds available from the lottery to be spent on food research. They will have to argue the case for the money being spent on their area of expertise.

HOW TO PLAY : Each team is invited on to the programme in turn. Their interview should last only about two to three minutes. They are asked to bring examples of their food category on to the show and are asked questions, e.g. *Why should you get the money for your research? Why is meat so important? Where does it come from?* At the end the group can take a vote on who should be awarded the money. The video can be copied and they can take their copies home.

Figure 4.15 Talking practice: 'Chat-show expert' scenario (taken from Rinaldi, 1998).

Following on from the social problem-solving activity described in the previous section, 'problematic' scenarios (e.g. taking faulty goods back to shops) can be acted out to enable students to practise assertive patterns of communication with staff before attempting them in real-life contexts.

Talking practice also provides a useful opportunity for students to develop monitoring skills and to give constructive feedback to each other. For example, after the practice students can be asked to comment on how they did; this feedback can be in the form of a gesture (thumbs up/ so-so hand signal), a score (points out of 5) or words (good/ OK/not so good). A written record can be kept of the students' monitoring.

Carryover tasks. Practitioners frequently report that one limitation of specialist teaching/therapy programmes is that they do not enable children to generalize their use of language outside the context in which it is taught. That is, children may develop a use of language in the formal teaching/therapy session, but fail to transfer skills to everyday situations where they need to use them.

The first point to make here is that children will gain from the positive experience of success, even if it occurs only in the formal sessions: success in a single context is better than no success at all. However, clearly, the lack of transfer to learning or communicative contexts is a serious limitation to teaching/therapy effectiveness and needs to be specifically addressed. The involvement of others who communicate with the child at home and school will be important here: this point will be taken up in the next chapter. However, the metacognitive approach does enable the children themselves to take some responsibility for the transfer of skills.

The teacher/therapist first needs to help children to become aware of other times when they can use a particular language skill and how this will be helpful to them. Poster material can be used to act as reminders at home and school, for example in other classrooms, assembly hall, dining room and, if the posters are laminated, in the playground.

Carryover tasks can also be set for each child. These will require them to use the particular skill they have been learning about in the language-focused lessons (e.g. a vocabulary set, a grammatical marker, a phonemic contrast, an interaction skill) at a specified time. A time needs to be chosen when a member of staff involved in the language-focused teaching is available to remind, monitor and give feedback to the child on completion of the task. Examples include an activity in another lesson, lunchtime (requesting food choices/talking to peers at the table), registration, etc.

The 'three steps' process described earlier in this chapter and incorporating activities listed in this section, is illustrated by the three examples in Figure 4.16

Example 1
STEP 1. Identify the language/communication skill to teach: grammatical marker plural 's'
STEP 2. Identify the curriculum subject in which to teach the skill: English (speaking/writing)
STEP 3. Develop an activity sequence with a build to learning from comprehension to use:

1. Comprehension
   i. Story: 'Sam's problem' (character who forgets to mark plural 's')
   ii. Poster: Don't forget: 's' means more than one!
   iii. Communication model: (script developed where speaker initially forgets to mark plural 's', e.g. asks for cup instead of cups. Listener only gets one cup. Child identifies and corrects the mistake; model repeated this time with correct use of plural 's')
2. Use
   i. Pairs card game
   ii. Hiding game: child has to find and name pairs of objects hidden around the room
   iii. Carryover tasks (speaking and listening/ writing)

(contd)

Example 2
STEP 1. Identify the language/communication skill to be taught: size dimensions vocabulary: LENGTH → long, short; HEIGHT → tall, short; WIDTH → narrow, wide
STEP 2. Identify the curriculum subject in which to teach the communication skill: Maths
STEP 3. Develop an activity sequence with a build to learning from comprehension to use:

1. Comprehension
    i. Story: 'Size magician' (gets size labels wrong; children laugh at him; he gets upset; they help him, etc.)
    ii. Poster: character demonstrating the size dimensions in humorous ways, e.g. eating long pieces of spaghetti etc.
    iii. Size lotto
2. Use
    i. Size dominoes
    ii. Quiz: children are asked questions about the size dimensions
    iii. Carryover tasks (measurement)

Example 3
STEP 1. Identify the language/communication skill to be taught: eye contact
STEP 2. Identify the curriculum subject: English (speaking and listening)
STEP 3. Develop an activity sequence with a build to learning from comprehension to use:

1. Comprehension
    i. Story: Looking Luke's story (Rinaldi, 1995) (described in Figure 4.8)
    ii. Communication model (poor eye contact → appropriate eye contact
    iii. Brainstorm (reviews "what is eye contact?"; "why make eye contact?")
2. Use
    i. Games: e.g. Come into my chair (described in Figure 4.12)
    ii. Conversation practice (child practises making eye contact in the listener role)
    iii. Carryover tasks (eye contact for speaking and listening across the curriculum/social times)

Note: some children will require a greater number of activities in the comprehension and/or use sections than included above

Figure 4.16 Steps 1, 2 and 3 of a language-based approach: examples.

Across the age range

The preschool period

In the preschool years intervention focuses largely upon the area(s) of language considered to be delayed or deviant in relation to developmental norms. Issues surrounding this notion were covered in Chapter 2. The difficulties in determining the specificity or full nature of the language difficulty in the preschool period were identified. It can be difficult to accurately assess children at this stage and as a result a number of education authorities have developed assessment nursery places in order to monitor children's development with the effects of formal education.

In the preschool period, the developmental model is used to determine the starting points and progression of intervention, from symbolic understanding/play and early interaction skills, to the development of single-word comprehension and expression, word combinations, phonological contrasts and so on. Although children have not yet entered school, it is important to consider their needs on school entry. In this way, intervention can be adjusted so that it prepares them for school life. For example, in phonology work, pictures shown to represent phonemes can be selected to reflect grapheme–phoneme correspondence which the child will later experience in spelling and reading work.

For example, traditionally, a gun was used to represent the phoneme 'k' or 'c' (hard 'c' as in cat, car, etc.): the idea was that the sound could be associated with the bang of a gun. However, it is now generally recognized that a more useful association in view of future literacy development is a picture of, for example, a car.

The development of basic listening skills is also essential for school entry, as is some experience of cooperative play and social communication with peers. These skills can be developed through structured group cooperative games, where the value of being part of a group is intrinsic to the activity. Two examples are shown in Figure 4.17; other examples are included in Rinaldi (in press).

Example 1: Magic Circle
A member of staff takes the role of 'magic fairy' and stands in the centre of the circle. A second member of staff carries out an action, for example, clapping hands or stretching arms or standing up. The fairy points to children in turn with a 'wand' and they must carry out the action. When all the children have taken a turn, a second action is shown – the children must then carry out this action when the fairy points at them with the wand

Example 2: Can you do what I do?
The activity leader carries out one or two actions (e.g. standing up and/or clapping hands) and then says GO! — all the children must copy the actions. The staff then show the children how it looks when they copy the actions together — at the same time. It's like they are looking in a mirror. The activity leader then repeats the actions and says GO! This time the children try to copy the actions together (this will be easier if they do them slowly). The activity leader then repeats the activity with different action(s).

Figure 4.17 Activities to promote group participation by young children. Taken from Social Use of Language Programme for Infants and Primary School Children (Rinaldi, 1995)

Perhaps one of the challenges of working with very young children is in capturing their interest against a background of often-fleeting attention and very limited understanding. Use of the visual modality is extremely important to hold young children's attention without being distracting. The author has found the use of intrigue an important ingredient in developing resources for this age group: the 'magic box' in which toys and pictures can be hidden is a particular favourite!

The principles of a metacognitive approach can be used with very young children, at a basic level. For example, Rinaldi (in press) has used the approach to develop early word knowledge and word combinations through animal characters. Not all of the activities described in this chapter will be suitable for this age group; however, a selection can be made in a way that retains the sequence of awareness/comprehension before use. For example, from the awareness/comprehension section: stories/drama sketches, pop-up posters, hiding/matching games; from the use section: simple game activities, simple carryover tasks. Metacognitive approaches clearly are more directive than other intervention approaches available to children in the early stages of communication development, such as non-directive play techniques (Allen, 1992; Tierney and Cogher, 1994). There is room for both types of methodology: children can benefit from the more experiential approach of non-directive methods as they can from a more conscious awareness of the process of developing language.

From primary to secondary school

When a child enters school, the developmental model still needs to be considered in order for them to learn new knowledge and skills; the importance of linking existing knowledge/skills to new learning has already been identified. However, a functionalist approach also comes into play, because it is important to look at what is expected of children both in terms of curriculum and social times.

In the main, experience suggests that the developmental model can be used in harmony with curriculum aims and objectives. For example, it is known that children learn first about the environment closest to them and find concepts relating to the 'here and now' easiest to grasp. This can be drawn upon in developing teaching content at each key stage. However, there may be occasions where it is necessary to step outside the developmental model in order to teach a strategy that will be useful to children. An illustration here is the strategy of compromise; a strategy that enables even young children to resolve conflict independently and provides an alternative to the child becoming upset when they cannot have their way. An understanding of the concept of compromise can require an appreciation of 'middle' concept, condition (what if we do X?) or consequence (let's do X and then we can do Y): these concepts are not a feature of early development. The author has found, however, that, using the metacognitive approach, it is possible to develop children's understanding of compromise, even at infant age, (labelled *things you do so you are happy and your friends (or mummy/daddy etc.) are happy*) (key words in bold). The concept can first be demonstrated and labelled in drama sketches (staff acting) and on poster material. Children then practise using the strategy with staff in acted out scenarios representing real-life situations (classroom, playground, home) in which they may need to suggest a compromise.

Experience suggests that at secondary school it is essential to retain a teaching model which enables more abstract learning to build upon existing/concrete knowledge. However, in some sense, there may be more conflict between the developmental and functionalist models in the secondary school years. It can be argued that, in some instances, applying a developmental model to teaching language/communication skills is less helpful at this age. For example, at the age of 15 years, students may achieve age-equivalent scores on standardized language assessments below 7 years. Applying a developmental model would suggest that it would be inappropriate to teach pragmatic comprehension skills to these children (concerning meaning open to interpretation) because such skills do not normally develop until the age of 7 or 8 plus (Bugental et al., 1970; Bugental, 1974; Ackerman, 1982; Cacciari and Levorato, 1989). However, in the secondary school years much of the language children are exposed to on TV, in reading material and in day-to-day conversation, assumes that they do understand these forms of meaning: plays on words, sarcasm, jokes, etc. Failure to specifically address these skills would set children at a considerable disadvantage. Using the metacognitive approach it is possible to develop an understanding of pragmatic meaning and thus prevent children being unnecessarily confused. For example, visual analogy and drama sketches can be used to demonstrate how context contributes to resolve ambiguity (Rinaldi, 1996).

Summary

A language-based approach enables children with special needs to access and retain learning. The key features of this approach are:

• Explicit teaching of a language or communication skill to have an impact on a broader learning or social target
• Multisensory methodology
• A framework to learn in graded, cumulative steps

The procedure starts by selecting a language skill/concept (for example, a phonemic contrast, a vocabulary set, a grammatical marker, an interactive communication skill) which will enable access to a curriculum subject (or aspect of social development). For each subject, the language skill/concept is then taught through an activity sequence, starting with awareness/comprehension and proceeding to use. Integral to this sequence is the application of the language/communication skill to a broader learning or social target. When children have mastered and applied the skill, the next is selected for that subject, and so the process continues. The relation between the different areas of language and curriculum subjects was covered in detail earlier in this chapter.

A metacognitive approach enables children to access even abstract concepts and can be used to develop skills and strategies of language, communication, learning and behaviour.

Appendix

Assessments

Boehm Test of Basic Concepts (Boehm) Psychological Corporation, Harcourt Place, 32 Jamestown Road, London NW1 7BY

Bracken Basic Concept Scale* (Bracken) Psychological Corporation, Harcourt Place, 32 Jamestown Road, London NW1 7BY

British Picture Vocabulary Scale* (Dunn, Dunn, Whetton and Pintillie), NFER Nelson, 2 Oxford Rd East, Windsor, Berkshire

Clinical Evaluation of Language Function* (Semel, Wiig and Secord) Psychological Corporation, Harcourt Place, 32 Jamestown Road, London NW1 7BY

Language Concepts to Access Learning (includes assessment picture book and profiles) (Rinaldi) Child Communication and Learning, 18 Dorking Rd, Chilworth, Guildford, Surrey

Metaphon Assessment NFER Nelson, 2 Oxford Rd East, Windsor, Berkshire

Phonological Assessment of Child Speech (Grunwell) NFER Nelson, 2 Oxford Rd East, Windsor, Berkshire

Pragmatics Profile of Everyday Communication Skills in Children (Dewart and Summers) NFER Nelson, 2 Oxford Rd East, Windsor, Berkshire

Renfrew Language Scales (Renfrew) Winslow Press, Telford Rd, Bicester, Oxon

Social Use of Language Programme Primary/Infant School Assessment (Rinaldi) Child Communication and Learning, 18 Dorking Rd, Chilworth, Guildford, Surrey

Social Use of Language Programme (includes assessment for teenagers) (Rinaldi) NFER Nelson, 2 Oxford Rd East, Windsor, Berkshire

Symbolic Play Test* (Lowe and Costello) NFER Nelson, 2 Oxford Rd East, Windsor, Berkshire

Teaching Talking (Locke) NFER Nelson, 2 Oxford Rd East, Windsor, Berkshire

Test of Language Competence* (Wiig) Psychological Corporation, Harcourt Place, 32 Jamestown Road, London NW1 7BY

Test of Language Development (Newcommer and Hammil) Winslow Press, Telford Rd, Bicester, Oxon

Test for Reception of Grammar (Bishop) published by the author at Department of Psychology, University of Manchester

Tests of Word Finding* (German) Taskmaster Ltd, Morris Rd, Leicester LE2 6BR

Test of Word Knowledge* (Wiig) Psychological Corporation, Harcourt Place, 32 Jamestown Road, London NW1 7BY

Understanding Ambiguity: An Assessment of Pragmatic Comprehension* (Rinaldi) NFER Nelson, 2 Oxford Rd East, Windsor, Berkshire

* asterisked assessments include standardized or comparison data with non-impaired children.

References

Ackerman B. On comprehending idioms: do children get the picture? Journal of Experimental Psychology 1982; 33: 439–54.

Allen C. In their own times. Nursery World Magazine June 1992.

Beattie L. Tips in Discipline with Children (4th edition). Aylesbury: Adlerian Workshops and Publications, 1996[3].

Bugental DE. Interpretations of naturally occurring discrepancies between words and intonation: modes of inconsistency resolution. Journal of Personality and Social Psychology 1974; 1: 125–33.

Bugental DE, Kaswan JW, Love LR. Perception of contradictory meanings conveyed by verbal and non-verbal channels. Journal of Personality and Social Psychology 1970; 16: 647–55.

Cacciari C, Levorato M. How children understand idioms in discourse. Journal of Child Language 1989; 16: 387–405.

Crystal D. Teaching vocabulary: the case for a semantic curriculum. Journal of Child Language, Teaching and Therapy 1987; 40–56.

Dean E, Howell J. Metaphon. Windsor: NFER Nelson, 1990.

Department of Education. English in the National Curriculum. London: HMSO Publications Centre, 1995.

Donaldson M. Children with Language Impairments. London: Jessica Kingsley, 1995.

Ehren B, Lenz B. Adolescents with language disorders: special considerations in

---

[3] Training courses are also available from Adlerian Workshops and Publications, 216 Tring Rd, Aylesbury, Bucks.

providing academically relevant language intervention. Seminars in Speech and Language 1989; 10: 192–204.

Guilford A. Language disorders in the adolescent. In Lass N, McReynolds L, Northern J, Yoder D (eds) Handbook of Speech-Language and Pathology. Toronto: BC Decker, 1988.

Kelly A. Talkabout: A Social Communication Skills Package. Oxford: Winslow Press Ltd, 1996.

Mitchell JE. Mastering Memory (manual and software). Sutton: Communication and Learning Centre, 1998.

Moats LC, Lyons G. Wanted: teachers with knowledge of language. Topics in Language Disorder 1996; 16 (2): 73–86.

Popple J, Wellington W. Collaborative working within a psycholinguistic framework. Child Language, Teaching and Therapy 1996; 12 (1): 60–70.

Rinaldi WF. The Social Use of Language Programme. Windsor: NFER Nelson, 1992.

Rinaldi WF. The Social Use of Language Programme – Primary and Infant School. Guildford: Child Communication and Learning, 1995.

Rinaldi WF. Understanding ambiguity. An Assessment of Pragmatic Meaning Comprehension. Windsor: NFER-Nelson, 1996.

Rinaldi WF. The Social Use of Language Programme – Storypacks for Secondary School and College Students. Guildford: Child Communication and Learning, 1997.

Rinaldi WF. Language Concepts to Access Learning. Guildford: Child Communication and Learning, 1998.

Rinaldi WF. Language Choices. Guildford: Child Communication and Learning, 1999.

Rinaldi WF. Developing Language. A Metacognitive Approach to Teaching Grammar and Meaning in Early Stages of Development. Windsor: NFER Nelson, in press.

Rogers B. Behaviour Recovery: A Whole School Programme for Mainstream Schools. Harlow: Longman Press, 1994.

Rogers B. 'You know the Fair Rule'. Strategies for Making the Hard Job of Discipline and Behaviour Management in School Easier (2nd edition). London: Pitman Press, 1998.

Rustin L, Kuhr A. Social Skills and the Speech Impaired. London: Whurr Publishers Ltd, 1989.

Tierney K, Cogher L. Non-directive therapy before school. In Law J (ed) Before School: Approaches to Intervention with Preschool Language-impaired Children. London: AFASIC, 1994.

Chapter 5
Implementing a language-based approach

WENDY RINALDI

Introduction

The previous chapter described a language-based approach; the focus of this chapter is on how to implement this approach in mainstream and special school settings.

The first section deals with a number of concepts and issues that need to be considered prior to implementation in any school setting. These are: a) collaborative practice between language specialists and subject/class teachers; b) the notion of a continuum of learning and c) inclusion (in contrast to integration). The chapter then focuses upon the special school and mainstream contexts, including the presentation of a model of inclusive education for language impaired children. A final section includes the different considerations pertinent to primary and secondary schools and the role of families in implementation.

As in previous chapters, the term language impairment is used to refer to children with specific language difficulties (including pragmatic disorder) and to children whose language difficulties form part of a broader picture of special educational needs.

Implementing a language-based approach: issues and concepts

Who does what? The language specialist and subject specialist

Language specialists

For the purpose of this book a language specialist is defined as a professional with a working or training background in language impairment. An assumption is made that such professionals are fully knowledgeable with regard to the needs of language impaired children.

Language specialists in education are likely to be drawn from the teaching, educational psychology or speech and language therapy professions. At the time of writing there are no formal training requirements for a teacher to enter the field of language impairment. Currently, the situation is that teachers tend to learn 'on the job' through hands-on experience with language impaired children, collaborative practice with other language specialists and postgraduate training courses. There are a number of university departments and other organizations providing short courses on various aspects of language impairment, listed at the end of this chapter. These are available to teachers, teaching assistants, educational psychologists and speech and language therapists (SLTs) and provide an opportunity for professionals across disciplines to learn together. 'Joint training' has been identified as an important element in the development of collaborative practice (Wright, 1996; Roux, 1996). Some postgraduate accredited courses for teachers are also listed at the end of the chapter.

SLTs undertake an initial degree course of three to four years, covering all aspects of human communication development and disorder. Regular updating post-qualification to allow continuing education and professional development is specified within the profession's standards, Royal College of Speech and Language Therapists (RCSLT) (1996). Educational psychologists study child development as part of their initial psychology degree and as part of their teacher training. There is some training on language assessment and strategies for supporting children with language difficulties as part of the professional training (Masters degree). Thereafter the amount of training can depend upon interest/professional development or be determined by the needs of the caseload.

Much of the research into collaborative practice with language impaired children has focused upon SLTs and teachers. The importance of SLTs and teachers working together with school-aged language impaired children is recognised and endorsed by SLT and teaching professions. (RCSLT, 1996; Ofsted, for example, 1996, 1997). Speech and language therapy for school-aged children could be seen as integral to the curriculum; ways in which this integration may be achieved were discussed in Chapter 4. The proposal of this book is for speech and language therapy to be timetabled as contributing to curriculum subjects.

The RCSLT makes reference to these kinds of considerations in setting out professional standards for SLTs working in mainstream and special schools: 'It is essential that a speech and language therapist in a mainstream school acknowledges her/his role as a member of the mutidisciplinary team. Intrinsic to service delivery in a mainstream school is the acknowledgement of the primacy of the child's educational needs.' (RCSLT, 1996, p. 56). RCSLT (1996) makes further reference to speech and language therapy being incorporated into the planning of the language programme in the context of the broad curriculum.

Wright (1996) found that SLTs and teachers working in specialist language units were able to identify many benefits from collaborative practice for the professional, including mutual support and the development of new knowledge. The latter benefit was reported more by teacher/therapist pairs based in the same school than by pairs where the teacher was based in a school and the therapist in a health clinic. Collaborative practice also creates considerable benefits for the child if language-based work is integral to broader learning experiences, as described in Chapter 4, for example. However, a number of potential problems have been identified which can create barriers to collaborative practice. For example, Wright (1996) notes that problems can emerge because SLTs and teachers are employed by different statutory bodies. Rinaldi (1998) refers to the importance of speech and language therapy services in education being managed by therapists who understand about working in schools. For example, teachers can feel uncomfortable when they hear of children being referred to as 'clients' or 'patients'; it can be very inhibiting for all concerned if the SLT has to attend meetings during child contact time: these kinds of timetabling constraints do not affect SLTs working fulltime in health settings.

Developing collaborative practice essentially requires *explicit* recognition of the complementary roles of all concerned (Beveridge, 1993). Roux (1996) suggests that the tendency for SLTs to be considered 'expert' may be limiting to collaborative practice because collaborative practice presumes an equality between professionals. Indeed, Wright (1996) found a two-way learning process between the teachers and therapists in her study. Teachers reported learning more about language impaired children's skills and needs; therapists reported learning, for example, about group behaviour/management and reading schemes.

Flemming et al. (1994) state that the different training backgrounds of teachers and therapists may lead to different perspectives on language. Experience suggests that teachers and therapists tend to have different starting points in considering the needs of language impaired children. The teacher may look to the curriculum for their starting point with the aim of giving language impaired children the same learning opportunities and experiences as non-language impaired children across the subject areas. SLTs may use their knowledge of the child's language/communication skills as their starting point and be concerned that children may not be able to make use of some of the learning experiences proposed by the teacher because of their language difficulties. SLTs, and other language specialists, may consider a developmental model in producing therapy programmes, which, as identified in Chapter 4, may not always complement curriculum objectives. An important point to make here is that, although the starting points may differ, it is not true that *never the twain shall meet*. In fact, the convergence of starting points can provide the optimum learning experiences for the child. It is possible, as described in Chapter 4, to teach curriculum subjects in a way that takes into account the underlying language difficulties. In order for this approach to be implemented successfully there needs to be an understanding of the subject area *and* the language needs of the children. Wright (1996) found that teachers and therapists were more aware of the differences between their professional roles than the similarities between them. However, it may be through the increased knowledge about similarities that they can establish a more efficient way of working. Indeed there is some evidence in the literature of a trend towards a convergence of approach. For example Miller (1999) urges SLTs to take greater account of social and educational perspectives and identifies speech and language therapy practice which has aimed to enhance curriculum success. Feiler and Gibson (1999) urge teachers to become more analytical in their approach, in particular, to evaluate the reasons why individual children might be struggling to read. Wedell (1995) refers to the importance of considering environmental factors (level of parental support, teacher expectation, etc.) and factors concerning the child's knowledge and skills (phonemic awareness, memory strategies, contextual comprehension etc.) in making this evaluation.

Wright (1992) found that collaboration is often attempted at the intervention stage with limited collaboration at the planning stage. However, Rinaldi (1991) identifies joint planning as a key factor in successful collaborative practice. The planning of a lesson creates a sense of 'ownership'; if there is not a feeling of joint ownership, one member of staff begins to feel at best secondary and at worst 'a spare part'. Further, the contribution a language specialist can make to a child's learning can best be understood and valued through the planning process. Rinaldi's experience, however, is that opportunities for joint planning can easily be eroded because it tends to be given low priority. In an approach based on collaborative practice, there needs to be a shift of priority here. Rinaldi recommends timetabling regular joint planning sessions to ensure that they do take place. Daines' (1991) concept of primary and secondary roles sheds further light on why collaborative practice can sometimes run into difficulty. In particular, this concept has current validity in exploring mismatches in expectation between teachers and SLTs. He reflects upon the changing roles of educational psychologists and notes some similarities in the ways in which speech and language therapy is evolving in some areas. He writes:

> Educational psychologists once used to have primary roles; that is, we would find a problem and try to do something about it ourselves through counselling, therapy or teaching. Now we largely support (secondary role). This does not mean that we get other professionals to do things to reach our objectives, though we are inclined to forget this.

Daines suggests that it is those in a primary role who have the final say over what is done and when. In this sense those in a supportive or advisory role cannot expect equality. Daines notes that SLTs sometimes support and are sometimes primary, and that this makes their teamwork complex and difficult. He observes that sometimes SLTs give advice to teachers that 'sounds as if they have simply written down their own therapy goals', which is not appropriate in a team context where the SLT is in a supportive role.

Clearly the area of collaborative practice is potentially complex and takes time to evolve. Sadler (1991) refers to the ultimate aim as 'two or more disciplines integrating their knowledge to produce new patterns of thought'. This aim may be achieved by some teams, however for others 'team practice may be at best a rather unsatisfactory parallel approach, or worse still, one in which there is little equality'. Perhaps a realistic perspective is not to expect an integrated approach from the outset. A number of stages may need to be reached as the team or partnership develops; for example the parallel phase described by Sadler may be a step towards a more integrated approach. The model outlined in Figure 5.1 encapsulates the development of 'the team' as an evolutionary process.

---

1. Feelings are avoided. Objectives are uncertain. The individual with primary responsibility takes the lead.
2. Issues are faced more openly, listening develops rapidly.
3. Personal interaction is established on a co-operative basis, the task is clarified, objectives agreed and tentative practices planned and/or implemented.
4. Feelings are open, a wide range of options considered, working methods are methodical, leadership style is contributory, individuals are flexible and the team is born.

Figure 5.1 The team as an evolutionary process (Daines, 1991; adapted from Woodcock, 1979).

The process of developing a team will be helped by joint planning, not only at the grass roots level but also at the school development level. Wright (1996) noted in her study that none of the interviewees worked in a school where there was a written policy about collaborative working practices. Rather, in most cases the teacher and SLT were left to sort out for themselves the way they worked. However, experience suggests that the best time to sort out how professionals across disciplines work together is not at the time when they are trying to teach children. Often professionals are expected to get to grips with the kinds of issues outlined in this chapter with completely inadequate preparation. Without sufficient preparation at the planning stages there is a possibility that misunderstandings or faulty perceptions of role may arise, creating a difficult atmosphere in which to work, and teaching/therapy which may not be complementary or, at worst, conflicting. If teaching and therapy presents diverse learning content this has the potential of creating learning overload and may actually be detrimental to the child's progress. Although teamwork clearly develops and fine tunes as professionals work together with the children, experience suggests that the foundations for collaborative practice are best agreed as part of the school development plan. When this takes place, teachers and SLTs have a sense of how, when and where they will work together before the children come to school. This agreement can also take into account whether the SLT is to work in a primary or supportive role. The process can then be developed further as the team evolves.

In this section the focus has been on how language specialists from different professional backgrounds work together. However, many of the issues covered also relate to team practices with another key player in the successful implementation of a language-based approach: the subject or class teacher. Collaborative practice between subject and language specialist is the consideration of the next section.

Subject specialists[1]

Subject specialists have a good knowledge of their subject and their priorities in terms of developing an extended knowledge of that subject area may not always coincide with the language needs of the children. For example, a Science specialist may plan to cover the ways enzymes act in the digestive system, assuming that students have knowledge of food word categories and understand the concept/language of nutrition. These may be faulty assumptions. Similarly, a Maths specialist may plan to teach the concept of probability to students, mistakenly assuming that they understand the vocabulary and vocabulary associates relating to present and future time. The ability to take a language focus requires a shift in thinking on the part of the subject specialist which can be difficult to make. There is

---

[1] In secondary schools, the concept of subject teachers or specialists is straightforward. In primary schools, class teachers are expected to have a sound knowledge across curriculum subjects and for the purpose of this section will be referred to as subject specialists.

a training issue here, but it may be necessary to identify that for some subject specialists this shift in thinking will take considerable time.

In Chapter 4, the need to appreciate two aspects of learning was identified: the language focused element and the broader learning context. Any study of a subject, beyond a basic sense will incorporate the development of a specialized knowledge and may involve skills that actually fall outside the language area. Some of these may be practical in nature or subject specific: for example mathematical skills such as subitizing (the ability to judge quantities of sets without counting) (Grauberg, 1998; Butterworth, 1999), visual and fine motor skills for Design and Technology, gross motor skills for PE, practical experimentation in Science.

Language specialists, in particular specialist teachers, can be involved in both of these aspects of learning: the language-focused element and the broader learning. SLTs usually spend more time on the language-focused work but they crucially need to be aware of the broader learning experiences. Often the way in which language specialists work together to complete the language-focused element of learning is dependent upon the time and resources available. However, the crucial point here is that the language-focused and broader learning elements need to be delivered in a way that will be complementary. It will not be enough to provide the language-focused element only. Ideally language-focused work should contribute to a broader learning experience within the same lesson or within the same working week; otherwise it will have less impact.

The concept of primary and secondary roles (Daines, 1991) is an important one in viewing how language specialists and subject specialists work together. This concept was introduced earlier in this chapter, where it was suggested that equality of role depended upon 'hands on' intervention with children. Those who advise or support (secondary role) cannot expect equality, because ultimately it is the person or people in the primary role(s) who make the decisions. It is proposed in this book that *in order for language impaired children's learning needs to be met adequately, a language specialist must have a primary role, or a subject specialist must be trained to a level where they can be considered a language specialist also.*

The proposed primary role of language specialists has implications for the way in which speech and language therapy is provided, in particular where the SLT is the sole language specialist. There is a trend in some areas for the SLT to be more consultative in nature; in some instances the SLT's contact with the child is through assessment only. There may need to be a shift in practice in this respect to allow SLTs to become actively involved in intervention and to develop collaborative practices based on equality of partnership. There is some flexibility here, since it can be envisaged that the concept of primary and secondary roles (or 'doer', 'adviser', 'supporter') may not be mutually exclusive and may overlap. Experience suggests that the role of adviser is most effective when the advice given stems from 'hands on' experience with the child and that this promotes a more equal relationship between staff. Those in primary roles are likely to develop an expertise which will enable them to advise others in the team.

The combining of language specialist and subject specialist knowledge will be considered further in describing the model of inclusive education proposed later on in this chapter.

A continuum of learning

In Chapter 1, a relation was identified between specific or primary language impairment (in the written and/or spoken modalities) and other special needs groups, in particular: sensory impairment, autism/Asperger's syndrome and more general learning difficulties. It was argued that a language-based approach works not only for specific language impairments but for any special needs group where a language or communication impairment forms part of the special needs profile. This is so because language can provide a 'window' into learning, because it can be manipulated. Concepts can be broken down and built up using simplified and then more complex vocabulary; words and word sequences can be demonstrated visually through action and picture. It was, however, acknowledged that children who do not have specific language difficulties may not see a language specialist and the curriculum, even in a special school, may not be modified in terms of a language focus; there is a training requirement here.

There is also a learning continuum between special needs and mainstream education. This point was indicated by the Warnock Report (1978), which stated 'the purpose of education for all children is the same; the goals are the same. But the help that individual children need in progressing towards them will be different'.

Specialist education has a great deal to offer mainstream teaching, because many learners benefit from the kinds of approaches advocated for children with special needs. For example, it can be envisaged that it is easier for all children to learn through multisensory teaching because students are more likely to be motivated if they become actively involved, and are more likely to remember teaching which has been visual, particularly if humour is used. All students can get a better sense of learning if they can see some kind of logical progression. Indeed children are often able to see this for themselves (Vaughn et al., 1993). Sebba et al. (1996) summarize the student's viewpoint well: 'We learn best when there are different things to do like talking, working in groups, drama, or other things, not just writing or listening to the teacher or doing worksheets all the time' (p. 16).

The continuum between special needs and mainstream education assists the process of children with special needs working alongside 'non-impaired' peers since a number of children who do not have statements of special needs may benefit from learning through a language-based approach. Indeed, Wedell (1995) emphasizes the diversity of learning needs and styles in all children: 'if an education system is geared to meeting the diversity of pupil's learning needs, the inclusion of pupils with SEN [special educational needs] becomes just one part of this diversity' (p. 101). The concept of inclusion is the focus of the following section.

The concept of inclusive education

Sebba and Sachdev (1997) summarize the difference between integration and inclusion.

> When pupils are *integrated* they may arrive with an individual programme or one is developed, which modifies or adapts the curriculum to increase access for them, often involving specified amounts of learning support from a teacher, or more usually a classroom assistant. *The organization and curricular provision for the rest of the school population remains essentially the same as it was prior to the pupil's arrival.*

Wedell (1995) emphasizes the point that integration superimposed on existing education is not what one is looking for in any attempt to introduce inclusive education. Rather, the process of developing *inclusive education* involves the whole school in *reconsidering and restructuring the organizational and curricular provision* to take account of the full range of needs experienced by the pupils in their community. The arrival of pupils with specific disabilities may challenge teachers to review the current range of teaching strategies (Sebba and Sachdev, 1997).

The language-based approach provides a method of restructuring curricular provision, which may be applied within the context of the National Curriculum. The model presented in the following section includes proposals for organizational restructuring.

A further issue is whether the concept of inclusion invalidates the existence of special schools. Some authors equate inclusion with 'mainstreaming'. Forest and Pearpoint's view (1992), for example, is that people can be included or not included but cannot be described as partially included. However, Sebba and Sachdev (1997) note that integration is sometimes used to describe arrangements for pupils that involve links between special schools and mainstream schools. This arrangement would appear to offer an intermediate stage for a transition from special school to mainstream education. It provides a useful dimension to the process of inclusion for those pupils who may need to start their education in a special school because of severity of need, but who at some point will be able to access a mainstream experience. However, an arrangement of this kind could only be considered towards a process of inclusion if the mainstream education on offer was sufficiently restructured and reorganized to meet the student's needs prior to transition. An important factor in the restructuring and reorgaizing of mainstream schooling will be in the training of mainstream staff. It would appear reasonable to assume that special school staff may have some contribution to make in this process.

Wedell (1995) notes that the more education systems have moved in a direction to give children with disabilities or difficulties an equal access to participate in society, paradoxically the more they have become entangled in procedures which tend to set special needs pupils apart. For example 'supporting pupils with SEN in the ordinary classroom often led to their having a teacher or teacher's aid who became "velcroed" to them'. Practices may now have developed to result in a more effective management of the support teacher or assistant's role in the mainstream classroom; however models of integration in current practice often do not attempt to adjust the class or subject teacher's practices sufficiently and this still sets students with special needs apart from their peers. If class or subject teachers do not change their practices to enable children with special needs (and other children) to access learning, the support staff are required to provide the access. When support staff have to provide the access to certain children only, this tends to make it more overt. In addition, this is less efficient in terms of teaching practice because in effect the content has to be taught twice.

Positive peer perceptions are important in establishing inclusive education; students can be helped to appreciate and respect the learning diversity of all pupils, not only those with special needs. A metacognitive approach is particularly helpful here, because, as described in Chapter 4, it incorporates learning about the learning process itself.

Many professionals and parents share a vision in which children with special needs can go to their local schools with children who live in their neighbourhood and where they can take advantage of the facilities offered by mainstream schools. The challenge then is to enable children to have these opportunities but not at the expense of their learning needs. Care needs to be taken to enable children to access mainstream education in ways that do not make it obvious that they have special needs and thus set them apart from their peers. Equally important here is to develop a school ethos in which pupils accept and value their differences. These were the starting points for developing the model of inclusive education described in the next section.

Implementing a language-based approach in a mainstream context

A model of inclusion for children with language impairments

A mainstream school probably provides the most challenging context in which to implement a language-based approach. Some factors that contribute to the challenge are outlined below.

1) Mainstream staff, including head teachers, may not fully appreciate the needs of language impaired children. For example, children who have specific difficulties with language may give a superficial appearance of not having special educational needs. It was noted in Chapter 4 that it is easy to fall into the trap of assuming that children with specific language difficulties know more than they actually do. The children have a cognitive ability that enables them to develop compensatory skills which can 'cover up' their difficulties: they are therefore sometimes able to complete activities without understanding the underlying learning point. A full understanding of the needs of language impaired children and the need to make a shift in focus to a language-based approach may take some time.
2) Children may lack the social communication skills to effectively manage themselves during social times. They may need support to develop appropriate social skills with mainstream peers.
3) The aim to provide teaching to meet the educational needs of language impaired children without setting them apart from their peers may be seen as more difficult to achieve in a mainstream than a special school context, because there is a greater diversity of learning need in the mainstream context. However, if the restructuring of organizational and curricular provision is sufficient it should be possible to meet this diversity of need.
4) The size of a mainstream school is likely to present more of a challenge to language impaired children, who frequently have difficulties relating to spatial awareness and who may have difficulty in seeking and/or memorizing verbal directions should they become lost. Noise levels (for example when moving from one lesson to another) can be intimidating for some groups; for example, children with forms of autism may have difficulty here.

Taking these and other factors into account, the model outlined in Figure 5.2 aims to achieve inclusive education for language impaired

1. A consultation and training period for local education authority representatives, governors, head teachers and senior management staff: the rationale and implementation of a language-focused approach; impact on staffing, timetabling, accommodation, etc.

2. Process to plan the reorganization and restructuring of curriculum: key personnel: special educational needs coordinator, head teacher, curriculum coordinator, subject head, language specialist coordinator.

   i) In every subject (or it may be appropriate to look at year groups in primary schools) there is at least one teacher who will work with a language specialist and become trained to use and develop the language-based approach with pupils who need it in that subject. This teacher must essentially want to develop his/her practice in this way. The training is carried out by language specialists (teachers or SLTs) trained in a language-focused approach. Training of subject/class teachers consists in part of formal training through in-service training but also involves the language specialist planning with and working alongside the subject/class teacher. The subject/class teacher and language specialist share a primary role with the children. The long-term aim is for the subject/class teacher to develop a language specialism and to use both perspectives ('language' and 'subject') to maximize their teaching effectiveness.

   ii) Each subject is divided into language-focused work and broader learning experiences. The subject and language specialists are involved in both elements, supported by (an) assistant(s) where necessary.

   iii) Children's language assessment profiles inform which subjects they will need to learn through a language-based approach.

   iv) Class size will need to be monitored carefully. Child–staff ratios may be higher than elsewhere in the school; this may be needed, for example, if children have attention deficits.

   v) Children register with a tutor group as any child would in any mainstream school.

3. A preparation period allows specialist language staff to complete training in a language-based approach and to begin training subject teachers.

4. Implementation. A monitoring/steering committee oversees process development.

Figure 5.2 Summary proposal for meeting the needs of language impaired children in mainstream education.

children across the special needs spectrum. The paragraphs below examine the rationale for the proposals made at each stage of the model.

Stage 1
A consultative and training period for local education authority (LEA) representatives, governors, head teachers and senior management staff, including the rationale and implementation of a language-based approach and the impact of implementing such an approach, for example, on staff levels and training, timetabling, accommodation.

The first step in the process is with the training of head teachers and other senior school management staff so that they can take the lead effectively in reorganizing and restructuring the curriculum and the manpower to go with it. There will be funding issues here that need to be presented to LEAs and government bodies prior to and during this process. A useful dimension of implementation may be to start with first year intake (year 1 primary or year 7 secondary) only. This enables a staged approach to the required reorganization.

Stage 2
The process of planning the reorganization and restructuring of the curriculum. The key personnel involved in this process will be the special educational needs coordinator, head teacher, curriculum coordinator, subject head, language specialist coordinator (SLT and/or specialist teacher).

At this stage, aspects of practice are agreed and planned, including staffing, collaborative working practices between language and subject specialists, a training programmme (for both the language specialists and the subject specialists) timetabling, accommodation. The aim is to achieve the following elements of the model:

1) In every subject (secondary school) or year group (primary school) there is at least one subject specialist (subject or class teacher) who will work with a language specialist (SLT or teacher specialist in language impairment) and become trained to use and develop the language-based approach with pupils who need it in that subject. *This teacher must essentially want to develop his/her practice in this way.*

Initially, it is likely that a language specialist will be required for each year group, or in a secondary school language specialists may work in (a) particular subject(s) across year groups. After the first few years of implementation, as subject/class teachers develop a language specialism, language specialists may be able to extend their roles, for example in training/outreach to other mainstream schools, liaison with special schools, etc.

The model proposes that the training of subject/class teachers is carried out by language specialists who themselves have been trained in and are experienced in using a language-based approach. The training for subject/class teachers consists in part of formal training sessions but also crucially involves the language specialist planning with and working alongside the subject/class teacher. The number of subject/class teachers trained to deliver a language-based approach will depend upon the number of language impaired children in the school (that is, including those with specific difficulties in language and those whose language impairment forms part of a broader picture of special needs). There may need to be more than one group if the learning abilities are very diverse.

In any subject area (or, in primary schools, any year group) not all subject or class teachers will be required to develop a language specialism and thus a degree of choice is afforded.

The point regarding the subject/class teachers having a choice in developing a role of language specialist is highlighted, since the motivation to change practice has been found to be essential for successful implementation of a language-based approach. The long-term aim is for subject/class teachers to be able to use both a 'language' and 'subject' perspective to develop their teaching effectiveness.

2) Each subject is divided into language-focused work and broader learning experiences. The language specialist and subject teacher are involved in both elements, supported by assistant(s) where needed. The subject/class teacher and the language specialist share a primary role with the children.

3) Children's language profiles inform which subjects they will need to learn through a language-based approach: not all language impaired children will need to learn all subjects in this way. In terms of setting or streaming, if this applies, it is likely that children with specific language difficulties will learn in a middle set. Certainly, the language-based approach should enable children with specific language difficulties, who have around average performance IQs, to do, at least, reasonably well academically. Language-based classes for children with language impairments as a part of more general, substantial learning difficulties are likely to form a lower set.

4) Class size will need to be monitored carefully. Child–staff ratios are likely to be higher than elsewhere in the school. Language impaired children may require one-to-one or small-group teaching to overcome significant deficits in attention, auditory processing or comprehension. Experience suggests an optimum class size to be in the region of 12–15 students, with a minimum of two staff.

5) Arrangements to enable children to more effectively organize their physical space may also be considered; for example, the development of clear visual signs including picture symbols and colour coding certain areas in the school.

6) Children register with a tutor or class group as any child would in any mainstream school.

Stage 3
Preparation. Prior to embarking upon a language-based approach, training needs to be completed a) to update language specialist staff and b) to enable language specialist staff to start training the designated subject/class teachers. In addition all staff in the school should be trained in an 'awareness raising' capacity. This stage precedes the ongoing training identified in stage 2, which occurs as language specialist and subject teachers plan and work together. Additional training from outside agencies adds to this process of continuing education.

Stage 4
Implementation and monitoring. A steering group should be identified during stage 2 which will act to monitor and support implementation. This group will include staff delivering the approach, as well as management representatives from the school and other agencies, such as support teacher service, SLT department, LEA.

The model of inclusive education described in this section has been designed to enable language impaired children to get the education they need in a way that doesn't seem particularly different from any other child in the school. The biggest difference is likely to be class size, but initiatives to reduce all class sizes will narrow the difference a little.

As identified earlier in the chapter, the process is also helped by the learning continuum between special needs and mainstream learning. A number of children who do not have statements of special need may benefit from learning through a language-based approach and may attend some lessons with children who do have statements of special need relating to language impairment.

Finally, it is important to see any model of inclusive education as a process rather than a state (Sebba and Sachdev, 1997). The monitoring and support body can act to facilitate further developments, for example, a longer term aim may be to develop team teaching practices between language specialist subject/class teacher and other subject/class teachers.

Implementing a language-based approach in a special school setting

Many elements of the model presented in the previous section also apply to a special school context. There will need to be a consultative/training period (stage 1) here also, either to introduce the concept of a language-based approach or to update and perhaps formalize an existing trend toward developing a language focus in the curriculum.

Implementing a language-based approach in a special school also requires initial planning at school development level to agree collaborative practices, training needs and to timetable language-focused lessons integral to subject areas (stage 2). There may be a considerable training requirement (stages 3 and 4) if staff are not accustomed to viewing their pupils' learning or social difficulties from a language or communication perspective.

It has already been noted that a language-based approach will, in some sense, be easier to implement in a special school because the majority of pupils are likely to need this kind of approach. However, implementing a language-based approach across a school (as opposed to particular classes, as proposed for a mainstream context) could be seen as more difficult to implement. Whereas in the mainstream context there was a degree of choice as to how much subject/class teachers became involved in delivering a language-based approach, in a special school, all staff are likely to need to make changes to their practice; changes that may be difficult to make.

The concept and issues surrounding language specialist and subject specialist, discussed earlier in the chapter, apply to the special school context in the same way as they do to the mainstream context. The training element of the model presented in the previous section, in particular the role of the language specialist in training subject/class teachers through in-service training and joint working practices, can be used equally effectively in a special school. There is a shared aim in both the mainstream and special school contexts for subject specialists to develop a specialism in language also and to be able to use both perspectives ('language' and 'subject') to develop their teaching effectiveness. Since the development of a language-based approach is likely to represent a shift (or an extension of an existing shift) in a new direction for the school, a monitoring and support mechanism is likely to be needed (stage 4).

It has been proposed in this book that a language-based approach will enable children with special needs (and some children who do not have special needs) to learn more effectively; this proposal applies equally to a mainstream or special school. Further, if mainstream and special schools can incorporate a similar approach to teaching children with special needs, this will assist in enabling a smoother transition from special school to mainstream learning. This will benefit those children who need to begin their education in a special school because of severity of need, but who are able to progress to the extent where they are able to access mainstream, language-based learning.

From primary to secondary school

The model for implementing a language-based approach presented in this chapter has been designed to be applicable at both the primary and secondary phases. The most significant difference is that at primary school language specialists work chiefly with (a) designated class teacher(s)[2], in each school year, across subjects while in secondary school language specialists work with (a) subject teacher(s), in each subject, across year groups.

It is probably true that the secondary school provides more of a challenge in terms of implementation, partly because of factors of environment and partly because of factors to do with the impact of the children's language/learning difficulties on social and learning expectations at this age.

Factors of impact and expectations were discussed in chapters 1, 3 and 4; the point here is that it may be more difficult for secondary school subject teachers to incorporate elements of a multi-sensory, language-based approach. The factors that may contribute here are:

1) learning content becomes more complex and diverse as children get older
2) non-impaired children become more able to rely more heavily upon auditory inputs
3) subjects become more specialized.

There is likely to be a greater overlap between primary school class teachers' existing practices and those required in a language-based approach, so the transition to the new approach may be smoother. However, clearly, an important factor here is the flexibility and 'thinking style' of individual staff members.

Factors that promote the primary school as a more 'user friendly' environment for language impaired children include the management of a relatively smaller physical space and a greater consistency being afforded by the same teacher teaching across subjects. However, open-plan arrangements are likely to prove difficult for children with attention deficits.

The potential problems of a secondary school environment are not, however, insurmountable and factors which make a primary school environment more user friendly can be drawn upon at secondary school. For example, the proposals made in the previous section will help children to manage the larger physical space of a secondary school. The teaching of a language-based approach at secondary school through desig-

---

[2] The number of class/subject teachers involved will depend upon numbers of children requiring a language-based approach.

nated subject specialists will also enable consistency across year groups and facilitate more effective planning of cumulative learning from one year to the next.

Involving families in the implementation of a language-based approach

In their Principles of Education for children and young people with specific language impairments, the charities AFASIC and I CAN recommend 'Parents should have their views heard and acted upon, and be active participants with the professionals in the planning and provision of programmes'. There is not only a moral obligation, but also an educational value in giving parents and other family members the opportunity to become actively involved in the language-impaired child's teaching programme. In Chapter 4, the need was identified to focus teaching explicitly on the 'carryover' of skills to settings outside those in which the skill was initially taught. Families can play an important part in enabling children to extend the understanding and use of language skills to learning and social contexts outside of school.

However, the need for flexibility is paramount. The aforementioned AFASIC/I CAN document gives some pointers here:

> Parents, siblings and the extended family will all need support in changing their perceptions of disability and developing realistic expectations for their child. Siblings may need support and should be given the opportunity to discuss their feelings. Sensitive understanding of each family situation will lead to an insight into the strengths and difficulties and allow appropriate support to be offered.

It may be difficult for professionals to understand why parents may not feel ready to become actively involved in teaching or therapy: why they may, for example, fail to attend appointments or carry out home practice. Sensitivity to each family's situation is crucial here. There may be other pressing demands on the family which need to be considered. Parents may not be ready to acknowledge the extent of their child's disability. This acknowledgement may be particularly difficult in instances of specific language difficulties. In these cases the child may not appear to have particular difficulties and there may be a strong desire to believe that s(he) will 'grow out of it' without requiring specialist help. In the words of Center and Rose: 'It may be difficult to face up to the fact that none of our clients (or their parents) want to see us. The need to see a therapist [or specialist teacher] is confirmation of their loss'. Parents may need time before they can focus upon the gains their child can make through specialist teaching/therapy and to adjust to the pace at which the gains can be made.

Parents may also need a period of time to adjust their expectations of the professional. Difficulties with expectation may be more likely to occur in a health context, because here parents' expectations may be more in terms of a medical model, that is, the therapist (akin to a doctor) will offer a course of treatment to remedy their child's difficulty. The notion of a partnership approach may carry mixed blessings for parents with these kinds of expectations. On the one hand, parents may value a more equal relationship with the specialist to acknowledge the contribution they can make, and a *sharing* of knowledge and experience (the specialist has knowledge/experience relating to children with speech and language difficulties; parents have knowledge/experience of their particular child). However, a partnership approach also requires a more equal share of responsibility than may be implicit in a medical model.

With these points in mind, it is appropriate to examine some of the options that may be considered in offering a flexible approach to family involvement.

Some options for family involvement

Parent(s) carry out teaching/therapy programmes with regular guidance from a language specialist.

There are some therapy programmes that involve parents in a primary role, tutored and supported by a language specialist. For example, the Hanen Programme (Manolsen, 1992) enables parents to monitor and develop skills to promote more effective parent–child interaction in the early years.

Parent(s) observe, support and reinforce, on a frequent and regular basis, a teaching/therapy programme taught by (a) language specialist(s).

In this type of involvement, parents retain a primary role in that they are working 'hands on' with their child. Their feedback to the language specialist also contributes to the planning process. Their involvement is tailored to support a programme led by a language specialist who also has a primary role in educating their child. The parent(s) makes regular planned visits to the school to observe and participate in activities selected by the language specialist which they can then repeat at home, either on a one-to-one basis or in the family group. The language specialist also spends time with the parent(s) to explain how these activities contribute to the overall teaching/therapy programme. Home practice activities may include, for example, board/card games (to develop vocabulary or syntax), interactive communication games or stories (to develop an understanding of concepts underpinning language/communication skills).

Parents observe, support and reinforce a teaching/therapy programme led by (a) language specialist(s) on a less formal and less regular basis.

Family group sessions can be organized on a less regular basis, perhaps termly. During these sessions, attended by the language impaired children and their families, language specialists working with the children can carry out with the families some of the activities that their children have completed in the previous term. Other activities can be demonstrated through video. Ideas can be agreed for home practice; strategies can be suggested in 'take home tips' lists.

Parents and/or siblings attend small group courses led by language specialists.

Topics may include, for example, How language difficulties underpin behavioural problems; tips and strategies for managing 'problem' scenarios; friendship strategies, etc.

Liaison via a school diary, occasional visits, parents' evenings. Strategies can be communicated via 'take home tips' lists or poster material.

Although providing a relatively minimal level of involvement, this option enables parents to be aware of teaching content and the strategies being suggested for their child. It opens the way for parents to develop their level of involvement at some later stage.

It is important to acknowledge that whilst parents have an important role to play in their child's education, in an informal sense and as part of the formal educational process, they also have another vital role beyond that of education. This book strives to show ways in which learning can be made more accessible and enjoyable for children with special needs. By the very definition of their difficulties, however, learning is not likely to be the easiest of pursuits for such children. Parents and other family members can give children an important space to be valued as they are, to relax, have fun and to take a breather from the learning process.

Summary

At the heart of this chapter is the proposal for an inclusive model of education for language impaired children. In the model, language specialists work closely with subject/class teachers to implement a language-based approach, drawing upon knowledge of subject and knowledge of the learning/language needs of language impaired children. The language specialist essentially has a primary role with the children. In the longer term, subject/class teachers may also develop a language specialism and be able to use both 'subject' and 'language' perspectives to increase their teaching effectiveness.

The ways in which schools need to reconsider and restructure organizational and curricular provision in an inclusive process were identified as including the development of collaborative practice between language and subject specialists, the identification and provision of staff training, a policy for flexible family involvement, the management of peer perceptions and adaptations to physical environment. Crucially, the starting point is at policy level where implementation needs to be agreed, planned and prepared amongst various agencies (school, specialist services, LEA). The role of special schools in inclusion was also referred to.

It is hoped that the model proposed in this chapter will provide a way forward for improving the quality of choice available to children with special needs. Currently the model holds 'concept status' only; it is however, presented with an objective of conversion to practice and formal evaluation, in particular, to enable children to enjoy a positive educational experience, where they can learn to the best of their abilities whilst not feeling particularly different from any other child in the school.

Appendix

Postgraduate training: short courses for professionals working with language impaired children

Continuing Education, Dept Human Communication Science, University College, Chandler House, 2 Wakefield St, London WC1

Child Communication and Learning, 18 Dorking Rd, Chilworth, Surrey GU4 8NR[3]

I CAN, 4 Dyers Building, Holborn, London EC1

SENJIT, London University Institute of Education, Bedford Way, London WC1

Accredited courses for teachers

Centre for International Studies in Education, University of Newcastle, St Thomas St, Newcastle-upon-Tyne NE1 7RU (specialist module options include Acquisition and Development of Child Language; Specific Learning Difficulties: incorporating Communication Difficulties, Dyslexia, Dyspraxia and ADHD).

Centre for Professional Development and Information (in partnership with Kingston University, Surrey) Whitefield Schools and Centre,

---

[3] Workshops for parents are also available.

MacDonald Rd, London E17 4AZ

Child Communication Studies, Speech Science, University of Sheffield, 20 Claremont St, Sheffield S10 2TA (distance learning course)

School of Education, University of Birmingham, Edgbaston, Birmingham B15 2TT (distance learning course)

References

AFASIC/I CAN (undated) Principles for Educational Provision: Children and Young People with Speech and Language Impairments London: I CAN/AFASIC, undated.

Beveridge S. Special Educational Needs in Schools. London: Routledge, 1993.

Butterworth B. A Model of Speech Production. Unpublished lecture, University College, London, Psychology Dept, 1980.[4]

Butterworth B. True Grit (opinion) New Scientist, July 1999.

Daines R. Close Encounters. Proceedings from the NAPLIC Conference: Partnership in Practice , 1991.

Flemming P, Miller C, Wright JA. Sharing the load. Special Children, November–December 1994; 9–11.

Forest M, Pearpoint J. Inclusion — the bigger picture. Learning Together, 1992; 1: 10–11.

Grauberg E. Elementary Mathematics and Language Difficulties. A Book for Teachers, Therapists and Parents. London: Whurr Publishers Ltd, 1998.

Manolsen A. It Takes Two to Talk. Toronto: Hanen Centre Publication, 1992.

Ofsted Inspection Report: i.(1997) The Park School, Woking, Surrey. Reference no. 125461; ii (1996) Meadowbank School, Gabalfa, Cardiff, ISBN: 07504 18257

Rinaldi WF. All Together Now: A Multi-Disciplinary Approach in Developing Children's Language as Part of Their Educational Development. Proceedings from the NAPLIC Conference: Partnership in Practice, 1991.

Rinaldi WF. Perfect practice: working together. RCSLT Bulletin, September 1998; 557.

Roux J. Working collaboratively with teachers: supporting the newly qualified speech and language therapist in a mainstream school. Child Language Teaching and Therapy 1996; 12 (1): 48–59.

Royal College of Speech and Language Therapists. Communicating Quality 2: Professional Standards for Speech and Language Therapists. London: RCSLT, 1996.

Sadler J. Training Teachers for Work as a Member of a Multidisciplinary Team. Proceedings from the NAPLIC Conference: Partnership in Practice, 1991.

Sebba J, Sachdev D. What Works in Inclusive Education. Barkingside: Barnados, 1997.

Sebba J, Ainscow M, Lakin S. Developing Inclusive Education at Rawthorpe High School: Report of the First Phase of the Evaluation. Barkingside: Barnados, 1996.

Vaughn S, Schumm JS, Kouzekanani. What do students with learning disabilities think when their general education teachers make adaptations? Journal of Learning Disabilities 1993; 8: 545–55.

Warnock M. Report on the Committee of Inquiry into the Education of Handicapped Children. London: HMSO, 1978.

---

[4] Butterworth's model is included, with kind permission from the author, in Rinaldi (1997). A Study of Secondary School Students with Specific Developmental Language Disorders. PhD Thesis, held at London University, Institute of Education Library.

Wedell K. Making inclusive education ordinary. British Journal of Special Education 1995; 22 (3): 100–4.

Wright JA. Collaboration between teachers and speech therapists with language-impaired children. In Fletcher P, Hall D (eds), Specific Speech and Language Disorders in Children. London: Whurr Publishers Ltd, 1992.

Wright JA. Teachers and therapists: the evolution of partnership. Child Language Teaching and Therapy 1996; 12 (1): 3–16

Chapter 6
Information technology for children with language difficulties

JANET LARCHER

Introduction

Information technology (IT) is a feature of all our lives and if we believe what we read in the papers then IT, particularly in the context of the Internet, will play an ever-increasing role. All schools are now linked to the National Grid For Learning and lottery funding has been set aside through the National Opportunities Fund to provide training to every teacher in the country on the use of IT and the Internet in their teaching practice. IT clearly has a place in supporting the language development of children with language difficulties, whether these are general or specific and regardless of their origin and etiology.

Literature searches fail to provide a theoretical background to the use of IT in the support of language development. Most of what is written is at a descriptive level, detailing practical interventions and their outcomes and coming largely from undergraduate and postgraduate dissertations rather than full academic research. I suspect that speech and language therapists do not typically have access to computers for use with children in their everyday clinical practice and that the primary focus of teachers is literacy skills. The use of computers in support of the language development of children with language difficulties is an area that appears to have fallen between these disciplines and thus not attracted formal research. I also suspect that similar reasoning explains the much greater availability of software to support literacy development rather than language development per se.

Software written specifically to help overcome specific language difficulties is rare, other than communication and symbolic based programs to support children with severe expressive language disorders (e.g. *Dynavox*, *Talking Screen*, *Winspeak*). There is much that is relevant, however, and it would be very easy for a chapter like this to become just a list of software: to avoid this I have adopted two strategies:

1. I have grouped and discussed examples of what is available in the following categories: preschool, multi-component packages, using symbols, initial letter matching and sound blends, specific concepts, whole-word approaches, word prediction, reading text, word tasks and word games and personal organizers. A final section deals with the development of communicative contexts around the computer.
2. I have identified three open-content programs (very flexible programs that allow you to add your own language/vocabulary) which can be used in a variety of ways to support language activities and which can be used to make new activities in many of the categories listed above. These are *Clicker 4*, *Inclusive Writer* and *Writing with Symbols 2000*. These programs are described in detail in the Whole Word Approaches section.

Multimedia computers offer sound, animation, graphics (including digitized photographs), access to dictionaries, maps, books, art galleries and museums, through CD-ROMs and the Internet, and these features are very motivating to children. A therapist in a major assessment centre relates that the centre is considering the purchase of computers because parents regularly report that children can do tasks on the computer which staff in the centre are unable to replicate through their non-technological approaches. Staff at this particular centre have concluded that the colour, game format, animation and reward style of computer programs is much more motivating to these children than just adult praise. What must be made explicit, however, is that IT is rarely used to maximum effect in the context of specific task-oriented programs. Its efficacy is rather in the imaginative use of a wide range of programs designed for use in a diverse range of contexts. Drill and practice programs can be used successfully if they are well targeted and used frugally, otherwise the motivating effect of the computer is quickly extinguished.

Most children with language difficulties will make progress and gain from using the computer through imaginative use of software that is unlikely to have been written specifically for the use to which it is being put. It sounds negative, even derogatory, to say that there is no inherent value in any of the software, but there are few if any programs that the child will gain significantly from, in the context of language development, if the program is loaded and the child is simply left in front of the computer. *Success with IT lies in the context of its use rather than in the software itself*. I will return to this theme in the final section of the chapter, after considering each category of use identified above.

Tiny Tech – software for preschool children

The audiovisual features of the computer make it ideally suited for use with younger age groups, and there is much software in this category. Parents, or professionals encouraging parents to invest in these resources, must realize that children quickly become familiar with this software and the programs need to be changed regularly – which can involve considerable expense. I am frequently asked if there is a library of such software, but there are none that I know of – largely due to copyright problems. This software is not generally available in high street shops and readers are directed to the Inclusive Technology, REM and SEMERC catalogues as good sources.

Software in this category can be divided into at least three stages:

Stage 1 covers the basic action and reaction bond – cause and effect software

Stage 2 extends simple cause and effect in that a) several actions are required to complete an activity, such as building a picture, or b) actions are required to be more accurate or specific

Stage 3 introduces the child to making choices and decisions via the computer.

Stage 1 – basic cause and effect software

The simplest software involves the child making an action – a movement or sound – and observing what happens. At this stage the action should result in the computer presenting something bright and colourful that moves and is noisy! This should encourage the child to:

- pay attention to the computer screen until the activity ceases
- then repeat the action
- observe what happens next.

In this way, the computer can be used to help the child understand the basic 'two-way' pattern inherent in the communication process.

Using a touch screen is the easiest way for the child to make this mental 'connection' between a) the action they make: touching the screen, and b) the effect: the computer screen erupting into a frenzy of activity! Some software, for example *Speak Up!* will react to the child making a sound (this requires a microphone to be connected to the computer). If a touch screen or microphone is unavailable then a mouse or trackball can always be used, and in some instances the software can be set to accept the press of a space bar or switch. These devices are less satisfactory because the child can be distracted by the 'instrument' of the action (mouse, keyboard, etc.) rather than relating their action to the effect on the computer. In a sense the mouse or keyboard acts as a third party in the interaction process.

A few examples of software that fit the stage 1 description are : *Ghost Train* on *Touch Funfair*; *Pin Wheel* on *Touch Games 1*; *Wake Up* on *Touch Games 2*, (all set to 'touch anywhere' on the screen); *Magic Painting* on *Touch Games 2* (set to one colour); *First Looks Patterns* and *First Looks Things* (set to one step); *First Steps*; *Touch Here!*; *Anytime* and *Startit* on *Making it Happen 1*; *Blob* on *Blob 1*.

Stage 2 software

All the above programs, except the last three, can be used at stage 2, but here children would be required to be more accurate about where they touched the screen – on the target – or they may be required to make several actions to complete the task and get a response from the computer. Other software suited to this stage is: *Build It!*; *Kaleidoscope*; *Switch Suites*; *Buzz Off* on *Touch Games 2*; *Rockets, Annabel and Dasher the Dog* and *Honey Bee* on *Touch Games 1*; *Lucky Dip, Darts, Hoopla* and *Coconut Shy* on *Touch Funfair*; *Surprise* on *Making it Happen 1*; most programs on *Making it Happen 2*; *Spikey* on *Blob 1*; *Abrakadabra*.

Stage 3 software

At this stage the child is required to make simple choices and decisions. For example, a picture is drawn on one side of the screen and the child is required to indicate which of three options on the other side of the screen is the same. In a further example, the child selects an option to match a particular dimension of the picture (e.g. colour). Initially it is important to select simple presentations and choices should be between items that are visually very distinctive. As the child progresses then more distractions can be added to the presentation to develop visual search and visual discrimination abilities. Software suited to this stage includes: the remaining programs on *Blob 1*; *Blob 2*; *Sort and See* and *Brian's Bus* on *Touch Games 2*; *Memory Doors* and *Hectic Highway* on *Touch Games 1*; *Choices*; *Face Paint*; *Reveal*.

Many other programs could be included in this section. The choice depends greatly on the child's interests, what catches their attention and the primary focus of the sessions. The suppliers' catalogues listed at the end of this chapter contain many ideas and some offer a policy of sale or return within 14 days.

Multi-component packages

A number of multi-component packages, sometimes offering a complete generative grammar approach from birth onwards, have been developed in the USA to support language development. These have rarely found favour in the UK, for a combination of reasons – style of presentation, language used, and the repetitive nature of many of the tasks. One possible exception is a package called *Earobics*. This is a collection of six games developed by people from a range of professions in the USA to develop auditory and phonemic awareness skills. There are two CD-ROMs, one aimed at children approximately 3–7 years and the other at 7–11 years. The games on the first CD focus on discrimination of sounds, auditory memory, rhyming, recognition of sounds, blending and segmenting. Each game has a number of levels, the focus of which are made explicit in the preferences section, and the therapist or teacher can set the tasks to be worked on or leave the child to start at the beginning and progress through. There are full reporting facilities. While there are one or two Americanisms, they are not intrusive and the quality is high.

This is one program where the skills and practice routines are quite narrowly focused, but what it offers is relevant to children with a wide range of difficulties.

Using symbols, signs and pictures

For some children with language difficulties the use of signs, symbols and pictures, used singly or in combination, can support understanding, communication, access to the curriculum, and reading and writing skills. There are a number of structured signing and symbol systems available and the reader is directed towards more detailed works on the subject than it is appropriate to develop here: Literacy through Symbols (Detheridge and Detheridge, 1997); Symbols in Practice (BECTA, 1993); Signing and Symbol Systems (Communication Matters, 1999) (see Resources, at the end of this chapter). The Widgit catalogue also has a very useful initial guide as a centre pullout. In this context, however, it is appropriate to comment that just one or two years ago mixing symbols from different systems, in order to use the one most relevant or transparent to the user for each item, would have been considered heretical. Now it is not uncommon to see Rebus symbols and Picture Communication Symbols (PCS) in the same book or chart, together with digitized pictures of family members and familiar locations. With an increasing availability of symbols and software to assist in making symbol pages, books and charts (*Boardmaker*, *Clicker 4*, *Gridmaker*), this mixing of symbols to provide children with a set of symbols that is most meaningful to them is likely to increase.

Widgit Software has been working hard to increase the knowledge of symbols and their effective use in both adult and child communities. Initially the only symbol systems available on computer in Britain were Rebus symbols and PCS, and only a few programs could handle more than one symbol set. Now Bliss, Compic, Makaton signs and symbols, PCS and Rebus can be handled by readily available computer software and indeed most software can now handle all the symbol systems. Two of the most flexible programs that can handle symbols are *Clicker 4* and *Writing with Symbols 2000*. Both of these programs are useful in a variety of contexts and more details on their use are given in sections below. For more information on the full range of software that can handle symbols the reader should consult 'Symbol Software' (CALL Centre, 1998) (see Resources, at the end of this chapter).

Initial letter-to-picture matching, sound blends and rhyming tasks

Programs requiring the user to match initial letters to pictures appear in almost all software catalogues, although *Animated Alphabet* appears to be an all-time favourite. Individualized versions of this activity can be made with *Clicker 4*, and the task can be extended using this program to select only those items in a grid of pictures (or symbols) that begin with the target letter. *Inclusive Writer* and *Clicker 4* also provide opportunities for creating your own sound blend activities. *Inclusive Writer* includes one such task among its example files: used in conjunction with symbols, if two selected components form a word then a symbol appears above the word to confirm its existence and its meaning. If the sound option is included the words constructed – real and otherwise – are spoken. Extra resources can be purchased for use with the *Clicker 4* program – *Picture Dictionary, Phonics, Nursery Rhymes* (including listening, matching, rhyming and sequencing tasks) and *All My Words*. While the program *First Keys to Literacy* suggests literacy rather than language tasks, the use of sound and graphics makes this a useful program in both categories. *Oxford Reading Tree Rhyme and Analogy Activities* is another useful program that has stood the test of time.

Specific concepts

There are a very few programs available which have been devised to help the development of specific concepts. Those that are available include: *Opposites*, which works on big/little, up/down, hot/cold, in/out and open/closed; *Spider in the Kitchen*, which focuses on positional concepts – in/on/under, above/below/beside, in front of/behind.

Whole-word approaches

For many children language and literacy go hand in hand: work in one area supports the other. Whole-word approaches are literacy-oriented, but programs offering banks of words, each of which can be listened to before being selected for use in a piece of writing, are powerful tools not only in developing language and literacy skills but also in building the self confidence and self esteem so often lacking in these pupils. Four programs – *Clicker 4, Inclusive Writer, Writing with Symbols 2000* and *Wordbar* – are widely and successfully used. At first sight these programs can be categorized as word processors, but they can do so much more and are quite difficult to describe in a manner that does justice to the range of ways in which they can be used. The first three of the programs listed can also be set to use symbols as well as words, just symbols or just words. These three programs are open-content programs which can be used in many other ways (for example, initial letter matching and sound blends – see above). *Wordbar* has a presentation style more suited to secondary age pupils.

Clicker 4

This program is typically presented as a grid of words at the bottom of the screen with a word (and/or symbol) processor in the top half of the screen. This is illustrated in Figure 6.1 using a Quickfire, level B, Weather Topic grid.

The grid can contain words associated with particular topics relevant to various stages in children's learning: from animal names and sounds to 'pond life', dinosaurs, the Tudors and many, many others. Grids can be linked; for example, an animal grid may be linked to others dealing with baby animals, the names for groups of the same animal, animal sounds, etc. A grid of present-tense verbs can be linked to matching sets of past and future tenses; a grid of sentence starters can be linked to grids containing objects, actions, and sentence completions.

Word banks, accessible through the first letter of each word, are also always available. This encourages attempts at 'sounding out' and is further supported by a feature that allows the words to be automatically re-ordered alphabetically when a new word is added. It is very quick and easy to add to the grids or make them from scratch, and classroom assistants have become very adept at producing new grids on the spur of the moment to meet new situations and teaching needs.

The program allows grids to be of any size, regular or irregular, and backgrounds and text to be in different colours. Hence it supports colour

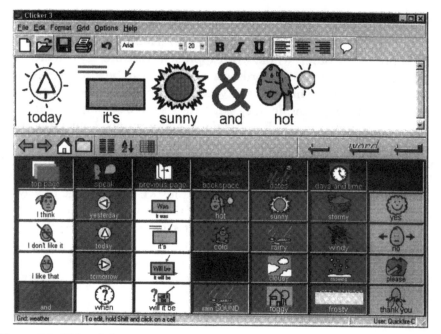

Figure 6.1 *Clicker 4* showing a Weather Topic grid.

coding for different parts of speech. Auditory feedback can be provided in a number of ways. The user can a) listen to the contents of a cell in the grid without adding it to their writing; b) have the cell contents spoken as they are added to the writing; c) have a keyword appear in the cell but a full sentence or phrase be added to the writing; d) listen to the sentence under construction at any stage or e) have a sentence read as soon as a full stop is added, or a paragraph read as soon as a new line is selected. The number of 'props' available to the user can be increased or decreased depending on the situation. These 'props', together with the fact that the text is directly in front of the user, seem to encourage the user to start on a task, to correct work and to achieve success.

Quickfire grids

These are a progressive series of four vocabulary files, using colour-coded PCS in Clicker grids. The top grid links to topic-oriented pages of vocabulary. The vocabularies gradually increase in grid size, number of symbols per grid, number of screens, and potential for sentence building. At all levels 'sentence starters' are available – i.e. whole phrases represented by one symbol (e.g. I would like, I'm going to, etc.) to reduce the number of

selections needed for sentence building. Each level includes the vocabulary introduced in previous levels. Workbooks are available for each level
and are intended to provide a structured approach to introducing the
vocabulary grids, and for recording responses. While these workbooks
have been designed for children with expressive language difficulties,
their structured approach and presentation style have led to success in
other contexts.

Writing with Symbols 2000 and *Inclusive Writer*

These two programs come from the same source – Widgit Software – and
there is intentionally a considerable overlap between the two. *Writing with
Symbols 2000* comes with 5000 Rebus symbols or 3000 PCS and the
support materials and examples are focused on symbol use. *Inclusive
Writer* comes with 2500 images, most from the PCS collection but supple-
mented by Rebus symbols and line drawings. The support materials and
examples are more word- and school-oriented and include rhyming words,
sequencing activities, story starters and word banks. Multiple windows can
be opened which 'talk' to each other, allowing word and phrase banks to
be created in one window for use in a task or in the other window.

As can be seen in the screen in Figure 6.2, users have a completely free
choice in their selections.

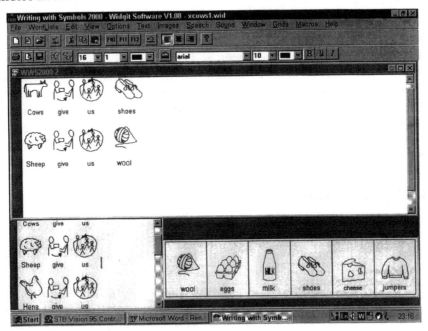

Figure 6.2 *Writing with Symbols 2000.*

One of the *Inclusive Writer* examples (referred to in the section Initial Letter-to-Picture Matching, Sound Blends and Rhyming Tasks, above) involves three windows. One window contains the sound 'ch', 'th' and 'sh'; another contains 'is', 'at', 'urch', 'ip', 'op', 'air' and 'ick' and the third is used to combine the two halves to form words. Another example includes one window containing the word 'Constantinople' presented as a series of letters, and a second window to attempt to form words from it. In both of these examples, as the letters are selected and sent to the 'work' window, the program confirms with a symbol or line drawing whether or not the word formed exists thus supporting word comprehension.

The spell checker also offers pictorial support, particularly useful for homophones (e.g. pear or pair). The program allows the user to look at the word in the sentence, hear it and look at the pictorial image. The graphical support for spell checking is obviously greater for *Writing with Symbols 2000* than for *Inclusive Writer* due to the relative size of the graphical libraries.

The content of the windows is easy to create and save as a collection of windows or 'environments', as the program calls them. Words, phrases or syllables can be listened to before being selected. Constructed text can be listened to at any time.

Wordbar

Wordbar can be likened to a mini *Clicker 4* program without the option of symbols and with a very non-childish presentation style. It is a toolbar which sits at the bottom of the screen and attaches itself to whatever word processor is used. It contains a number of banks of grids. Each grid can be of variable size and contain single words or phrases. It is quick and easy to add words or phrases to an existing grid or to create a new grid. Grids can be sorted automatically into alphabetical order. The screen in Figure 6.3 shows *Wordbar* being used to provide a range of adjectives for describing individual features.

Word prediction

Word prediction software runs alongside other word processing packages and attempts to predict the word being typed based on recency, frequency and rules of English grammar. It does this by offering a list of words which is updated each time a new letter is typed. As soon as the required word is offered it can be selected and added to the text. This approach can help with spelling since all words will be correctly spelt and it is easier to recognize the required word than to recall the correct spelling of a word. Some predictors allow the user to listen to the predicted words, which is partic-

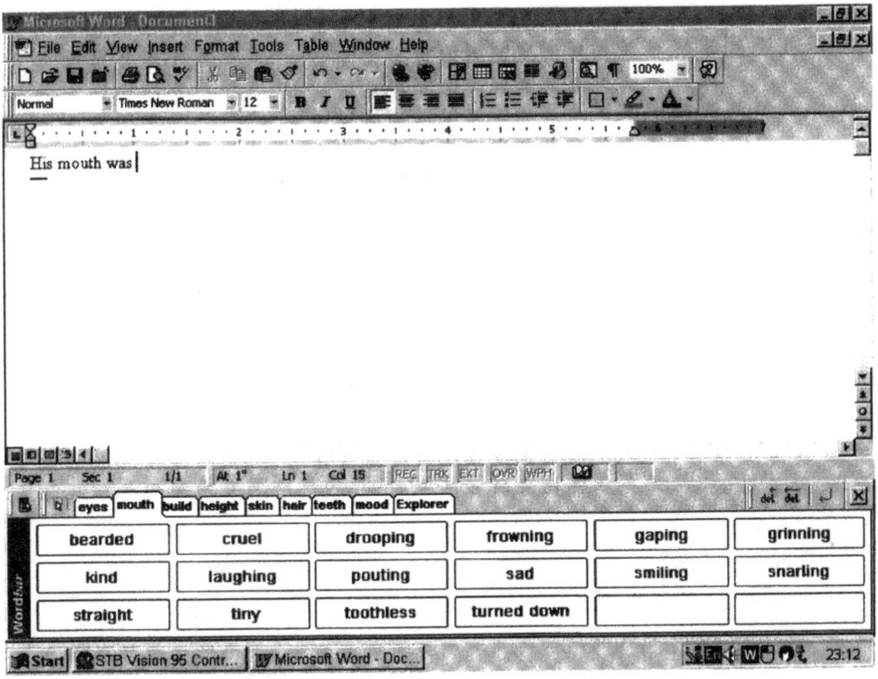

Figure 6.3 *Wordbar* provides a range of adjectives for describing individual features.

ularly useful when users are required to distinguish between words that are similar in appearance.

Since it takes a time to scan the list of suggestions, a helpful strategy is to teach the user to type at least the first three letters of the word before looking at the predictions – at which stage the required word will usually be offered in the prediction list. If they are using a full dictionary and no words are offered, they have probably made a mistake and should reconsider the letters that they have typed. Structured teaching around this approach has made this a workable and useful strategy for some pupils.

A dictionary can be constructed for less able pupils using a smaller number of words so that there is a high probability of their required word being predicted after just one letter. Such dictionaries are often based on the 200 most frequently used words, with other specific vocabulary being added as required.

A number of these programs are available and purchasers should ensure that the prediction algorithm is based on grammar as well as recency and frequency rules. Two programs that I have found to be particularly good are *Co-Writer* and *Penfriend*. *Prophet* offers a word morphology option, particularly helpful for children with language diffi-culties. Once the user has chosen the basic word, e.g. 'make', related words such as 'makes', 'made' and 'making' are also offered. Another program to consider in this context is *Read and Write*. While the predic-tion algorithm in *Read and Write* is not so effective, the program can read back text files or parts thereof (Reading Text, below).

Co-Writer

This program is different from other prediction programs in that it opens its own window in the bottom half of the of the word processor screen (as illus-trated in Figure 6.4), and the user constructs the sentence in this window before sending it to the main word processor. This approach allows a greater range of props to be used to support the writer, including colour of background, size of text, speech, number of options presented and whether they are presented below the line of text or in place within the text.

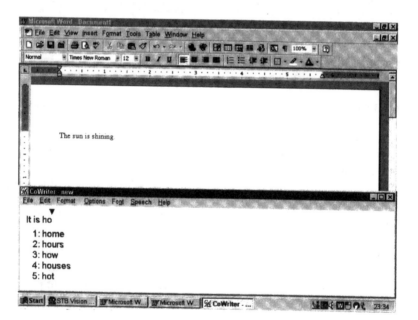

Figure 6.4 *Co-Writer* uses a range of props to help students form sentences.

Penfriend

This program opens a small window on the word processing page to contain the predictions. Within this window the colour of the background can be changed, as well as the colour, size and font of the text. The number of options can be increased by using a larger window.

Reading text

Some pupils appear to have good spoken skills but have difficulty with reading and writing. While some of the options already discussed will assist with writing, there are also programs that can read text to the user. Hence chapters from books, etc., required for homework can be scanned into a computer and the text files thus created can be read to the pupil. A number of programs are available to do this but the most easily available and widely used in a schools context is *Read and Write*. Another particularly useful program to explore is *Wynn*.

Read and Write

This program places an extra toolbar on the page that can be used to control the props offered to the user. A feature which is very popular with younger users (and many older ones!) is an animated wizard character that speaks the messages and text – if this option is selected. The program offers word prediction, a thesaurus and screen reading as well as options to: spell check as you type, speak each word as it is typed, change text and background colours, capture homophones and speak the meaning. This program probably offers the most features to support writers within a single program, but in my experience each of its individual features is not as good as programs that do only that particular task. For example, *Penfriend* is quicker to offer predictions and is more likely to offer the required word than *Read and Write*.

Word tasks and word games

The best-known program in this category is *Wordshark*. It provides 26 different games to emphasize word recognition and spelling. Other programs in this category offer cloze procedures (e.g. *Cloze* and *Sherlock*) so that the pupil needs to draw on their knowledge of language as well as of the world to predict what letters/words are required to complete a piece of text. Once again, this is a task that works well as a group activity, or in pairs or with an adult to encourage discussion and to develop topics that arise. Additional pictorial/auditory supports can sometimes be included.

Personal organizers

Pupils with pragmatic disorders find it difficult to organize themselves. Computers running recent versions of Windows come with a program called *Microsoft Outlook*. The calendar option can be used as a diary, but it also gives alarms at appropriate times if set. These pages can be printed, giving a daily schedule. This program, or others with similar features, is found on palmtop computers which are light and easy to carry around and therefore realistic to have permanently available to the user.

Creating communicative contexts around the computer

In the introduction to this chapter it was emphasized that success with IT lies in the context of its use rather than in the software itself. Many programs and CD-ROMs can provide a starting point to give a shared focus for looking, communication and language development. This type of use is only limited by the context setter's imagination, knowledge of computer use and availability of materials, although if the user has access to the Internet there are some wonderful materials – in amongst a great deal of dross! The *My World* program and its associated scenarios can provide a wide range of topics.

Many children love to play, indeed some would say get hooked on, computer games. However, collaborative play with computer games can provide an opportunity for children to apply interactive communication and language skills (such as vocabulary, word order, task sequencing, etc.) that they have been taught elsewhere.

The computer can also help make more traditional learning activity fun. For example, the development of class and individual pupil books offers enormous scope and infinite opportunities for shared communicative context around the computer.

Talking stories

Earlier in this chapter it was stated that there are few programs that work on their own to facilitate language development. An exception to this may be talking stories presented on a multimedia computer. A wide variety of these are available on CD-ROM – *Broderbund Living Books* being excellent examples. The precise features of each talking story vary, but in general the computer presents a picture with the story written under it in bold text. The story can be read aloud by the computer, each word highlighted as it is spoken, or the words can be spoken as the child points to them with a pointing device – mouse, trackball or touch screen. Many of these stories have interesting graphics, features of which can be animated by selecting them with the pointing device. While children will benefit from exploring the pictures and reading, or having the story read to them, a great deal more is achieved if the program is used to provide a shared focus with another child, the adult facilitating language/communication opportunities as appropriate.

Summary

This chapter has identified some of the ways in which computers can be used to assist children who have language difficulties. Software exemplars have been given for a number of categories of use and some open-content software identified which can be tailored to children's specific interests and vocabulary. Software in some of these categories teaches skills directly, while software in other categories supports weaknesses (e.g. reading texts). Some software could be used in both ways (e.g. word prediction). Future research may suggest that one type of software is more useful or productive than others. I hope that this chapter will give ideas and present some challenges to researchers in this field, as well as to therapists and teachers.

Resources

Software referred to in the text
Abrakadabra – Inclusive Technology Ltd
Animated Alphabet – Sherston Software Ltd
Blob 1 and 2 – Widgit Software Ltd; Inclusive Technology Ltd
Boardmaker – Cambridge Adaptive Communication; Don Johnson Special Needs; and SEMERC
Broderbund Living Books – Inclusive Technology Ltd
Build It! – SEMERC
Choices – Widgit Software Ltd; Inclusive Technology Ltd
Clicker 4 and associated resources – Crick Software; SEMERC
Cloze – SEMERC
Co-Writer – Don Johnson Special Needs
Dynavox Software – Sunrise Medical Ltd
Earobics – Don Johnson Special Needs
Face Paint – SEMERC
First Keys to Literacy – Widgit Software Ltd; Inclusive Technology Ltd
First Looks – Inclusive Technology Ltd
First Steps – SEMERC
Gridmaker – Widgit Software Ltd
Inclusive Writer – Inclusive Technology Ltd; Widgit Software Ltd
Kaleidoscope – Inclusive Technology Ltd; SEMERC
Making It Happen – Widgit Software Ltd
Microsoft Outlook – Microsoft
My World – Inclusive Technology Ltd; SEMERC
Opposites – Inclusive Technology Ltd
Oxford Reading Tree Rhyme and Analogy Activities – Sherston Software
Penfriend – Design Concept & Inclusive Technology Ltd
Prophet – The ACE Centre, Oxford
Read and Write – Iansyst Ltd; Inclusive Technology Ltd
Reveal – Inclusive Technology Ltd; SEMERC
Sherlock – SEMERC

Speak Up! – Sensory Software
Spider in the Kitchen – Inclusive Technology Ltd
Switch Suites – Inclusive Technology Ltd
Symbol Software – The CALL Centre
Talking Screen – Cambridge Adaptive Communication
Touch Funfair – SEMERC
Touch Games 1 & 2 – SEMERC
Touch Here! – Inclusive Technology Ltd; SEMERC
Winspeak – Sensory Software; Cambridge Adaptive Communication
Wordbar – Crick Software
Wordshark – Inclusive Technology Ltd; SEMERC
Writing with Symbols 2000 –Widgit Software Ltd; Inclusive Technology Ltd
Wynn – Don Johnson Special Needs

Suppliers

The ACE Centre, The Wooden Spoon Building, 92, Windmill Rd, Headington OX3 7DR. Tel: 01865 763508
The CALL Centre, Paterson's Land, Holyrood Rd, Edinburgh EH8 8AQ
Crick Software, 1 The Avenue, Spinney Hill, Northampton NN3 6BA. Tel: 01604 671692
Cambridge Adaptive Communication, The Mount, Toft, Cambridgeshire CB3 7RL Tel: 01223 264244
Design Concept, 30 Oswald Rd, Edinburgh EH9 2HG. Tel: 0131 668 2000
Don Johnson Special Needs, 18 Clarendon Court, Calver Road, Winwick Quay, Warrington WA2 8QP. Tel: 01925 241642
Iansyst Ltd, The White House, 72 Fen Rd, Cambridge CB4 1UN. Tel: 0500 141515
Inclusive Technology Ltd, Saddleworth Business Centre, Delph, Oldham OL3 5DF. Tel: 01457 819790
REM Ltd, Great Western House, Langport, Somerset TA10 9YU. Tel: 01458 254701
SEMERC, Granada Learning Ltd, Granada Television, Quay St, Manchester M60 9EA. Tel: 0161 827 2966
Sensory Software, 26 Abbey Rd, Malvern, Worcestershire WR14 3HD
Sherston Software Ltd, Angel House, Sherston, Malmesbury, Wiltshire SN16 0LH. Tel: 01666 843200
Sunrise Medical Ltd., High St, Wollaston, West Midlands DY8 4PS. Tel: 01384 446688
Widgit Software Ltd, 102 Radford Rd, Leamington Spa CV31 1LF. Tel: 01926 885303

Other resources referred to in the text

Detheridge M, Detheridge T. Literacy Through Symbols. London: David Fulton Publishers, 1997 (also available from Widgit Software Ltd)
Symbols In Practice, NCET 1993, BECTA, Milburn Road, Science Park, Coventry CV4 7JJ
Symbol and Signing Systems (free information leaflets) Communication Matters c/o The ACE Centre, The Wooden Spoon Building, 92 Windmill Rd, Headington OX3 7DR. Tel: 01865 763508

Index